COMFORTABLY INSANE

A JOURNEY FROM THE HELL OF ALCOHOLISM TO A HEALTHY PRODUCTIVE LIFE

NEAL LINARES

Copyright © 2019 by Neal Linares

Comfortably Insane

All rights reserved. No part of this publication may be reproduced, distributed or transmitted in any form or by any means, including photocopying, recording, or other electronic or mechanical methods, without the prior written permission of the publisher, except in the case of brief quotations embodied in critical reviews and certain other noncommercial uses permitted by copyright law.

Although the author and publisher have made every effort to ensure that the information in this book was correct at press time, the author and publisher do not assume and hereby disclaim any liability to any party for any loss, damage, or disruption caused by errors or omissions, whether such errors or omissions result from negligence, accident, or any other cause.

Adherence to all applicable laws and regulations, including international, federal, state, and local governing professional licensing, business practices, advertising, and all other aspects of doing business in the US, Canada or any other jurisdiction is the sole responsibility of the reader and consumer.

Neither the author nor the publisher assumes any responsibility or liability whatsoever on behalf of the consumer or reader of this material. Any perceived slight of any individual or organization is purely unintentional.

Some names have been changed to protect the privacy of individuals.

The resources in this book are provided for informational purposes only and should not be used to replace the specialized training and professional judgment of a health care or mental health care professional.

Neither the author nor the publisher can be held responsible for the use of the information provided within this book. Please always consult a trained professional before making any decision regarding treatment of yourself or others.

ISBN: 978-1-7334235-1-9

Cover Design by: 100 Covers

Edited by: Katie Chambers of Beacon Point LLC

Resources: www.comfortablyinsane.com

Dedication

To Zach, my amazing son, I sense your goodness every time we talk. Without you this book does not happen.

To Amy, my amazing wife, you're my partner, my friend, and everything in my life. Thanks for letting me be me.

This book is dedicated to anyone who is suffering with alcoholism or some type of addiction. Know that there's always hope, even if you don't believe.

If you're suffering and reading this, my best advice is to make it to a meeting. Become comfortable with the idea that you will find part of your solution there.

Your presence has helped me many times as I have seen you walk in with desperation. Know that someone is watching, and someone is being helped by your presence alone. Learn to say, "I need help!"

To everyone, I love you. I truly dedicate this book to anyone who might find strength and hope.

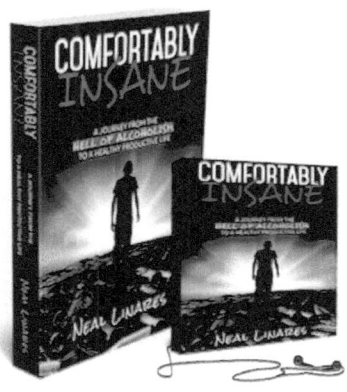

The Number One Question I'm Always Asked Is:

"Neal, Do You Have An Audiobook?"

For a long time I didn't! But finally now I do and the ONLY way to GET it is through this special offer.

Go to: audiobook.comfortablyinsane.com

"Transformation isn't sweet and bright. It's a dark and murky, painful pushing. An unraveling of the untruths you've carried in your body. A practice in facing your own created demons. A complete uprooting before becoming."

—Victoria Erickson, *Edge of Wonder.*

Table of Contents

Part 1: Laying the Foundation — 1

How It Started	3
The Beginning	7
The Betrayal	17
The First Night	19
The Good, the Bad, and the Beautiful	25
The Third Year	33
Military School Ends	37
Life After Military School	41
The Incident	45
Back in the USA!	47
The First Step	53
Welcome to Miami	57
The 180	65

Part 2: The Comfort of Insanity — 69

Eight Years of White Knuckling	71
I Feared Sanity	77
The Big Burst!	81
At the Bar	83
The Decline	87
End of Fantasy	93
Stop!	101
Hi. My Name Is Neal, and I'm An Alcoholic	105
Who Are You Here For?	111
I'm Sick	115
The Twenty-Year First Step	117
The Business and My Dad	119
Working My Recovery	123
The Blitz	127
Step Five and the Bus	131
Trudging the Road of Sobriety	139
I'm Cured?	143
Graduation! Happily Never After	151

Part 3: Trudging the Happy Road of Life — 155

The Legacy	157
Amber and Becoming a Lawyer	161
The Pattern	167
The Gift of Desperation	171
Stability in Chaos	173
I Count	175
He Made Me. Build on This Foundation	177
Back to Basics	179
The Move	181
Bliss	185
And Then There Was Amy!	187
Acknowledgments	193
Random Thoughts	195
About the Author	199

PART 1

LAYING THE FOUNDATION

How It Started

"Forgiveness says you're given another chance to make a new beginning."

—Desmond Tutu

It's pretty dark out here. I hear footsteps. They sound sloppy and unrhythmical, as if fruit were falling from a tree. I'm breathing heavily. Why am I so confused? I realize I am walking on a street that I drive through quite often, but why is it so dark? Why are my feet moving without my control? Why can't I think straight?

At a distance, I see red and blue lights and sarcastically think, *it's Santa Claus.* But wait; it's not even Christmas! I try to get control of my feet and find that I'm unable to. I try but can't!

I'm walking almost on autopilot but very determined, and, yes, now I remember; I'm walking home. But why?

As Santa's lights slowly approach, I start to focus and gain control of my body a little better, but not much. I try to quicken my step. But the heat—very typical of lovely Miami where people come to party, and I'm no exception—slows me down.

This moment in my life seemed to mark the start of a new beginning. It was the culmination of a life of pain and destruction and the beginning of a life full of peace and serenity. I guess it's normal for one phase of life to begin when another phase ends, but when you're not interested in phasing out the pain and destruction and, instead, are forced to do it, it feels as if you might die.

But before I tell you about the events leading up to this pivotal moment, let me tell you a little about me. At the time of this writing, I'm forty-seven. I attempted to write this book two years ago, but for many reasons, could not. I have felt it burning in my chest since 2009, probably even before that. Life has changed dramatically for me. Parts of this book I wish I would have written sooner. Nevertheless, things happen when they happen. I've learned there's always a reason for everything that happens, and it happens that now I'm writing this book.

I was born in SLC, Utah. It was a very nice place to live, although I realized that I've always been confused about life, and maybe it's because I wasn't the right skin color for my surroundings in Utah. My parents are natives of El Salvador. I once heard it best. I'm an American-born Salvadorian or Hispanic. So, in other words, I'm brown. Haha.

Yet, when I went to El Salvador, which was half my life back and forth until I was around 18, I never felt fully comfortable there either, so it was hard to determine where I was from sometimes.

Although several times while growing up I might have felt mistreated due to my ethnicity, I truly don't feel that has ever affected my development. People can just be mean. I don't think it's a USA thing or an El Salvador thing, as I've met the same type of mean people in both countries. In fact, I think I, myself, have been a jerk to other people at times; however, I know for a fact that the nice people far outnumber the jerks.

In the beginning, going to school in both countries seemed confusing, but I gelled in both. Maybe a bit more in El Salvador;

HOW IT STARTED

however, I did understand both cultures. That would be a good example of my life to come. I felt that I understood things and people and situations, but I was never really good at explaining what they meant or how they made me feel. Honestly, I'm not sure if that affected how I was and the transformation to understanding and experiencing joy. Before my pivotal moment, I often wondered, in the countless complete blackouts, what would have happened if I simply didn't come out of them and just passed on to the other world? Would I still be drunk? Or would all that go away? If so, then maybe the pain and rejection would leave as well. I truly thank God for not letting me find out. As I have discovered, there's so much to life. So much that I didn't know and so much that I've yet to learn.

It really felt as if I hadn't ever been able to experience joy in my youth. Yes, there had been some happy moments, but they were always riddled with self-doubt and misunderstanding of how I was supposed to feel or act. I still struggle with this sometimes. To give you an example, this book has been burning in my chest for a long time. There were times I felt helpless about this; however, I also knew there was something I could do about it and finished it. I can bounce between these two extremes obsessively. My life seems to be that way. I must either be on an extreme obsessive path to get things done or do nothing at all. This thought process has proven to destroy any attempts at being happy. Thus, the dilemma, the balancing act.

My theory is that we are all given the same set of basic human emotions. Love, joy, surprise, fear, sadness, anger, disgust, shame, pride. We all have them. Each one of us just has them in different proportions, or rather are out of balance with some. I think everyone faces this at different levels. The test in life is to learn to balance them.

COMFORTABLY INSANE

This is the story of my transformation from being an alcoholic to living a sober and happy life, not perfect, but calm. Although there's a lot to share about my parents' imperfections and even more to share about my parents' good and kind deeds, I won't focus on that. I've come to realize that I'm responsible for the way I've lived my life, and not them. To take this point further, no one is responsible for my mishaps. This concept changed my life and has kept me safe, whereas before, I would blame everyone else for all my troubles.

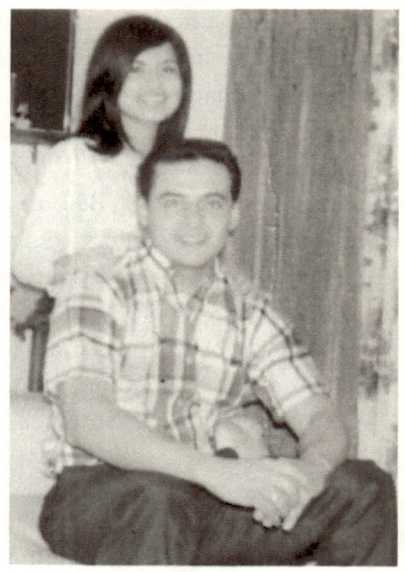

My parents as six month newlyweds.

If you, dear reader, are an alcoholic or addict, I hope that you find comfort and solace, or merely relate a bit to these words. Also, if you know someone suffering from alcoholism or addiction, this can serve as a perspective inside the mind of an addict.

> **Lesson Learned:** The doors of recovery are hard to recognize. Don't be afraid to knock and find out.

The Beginning

"A journey of a thousand miles begins with a single step."

—Lao Tzu

When I was a little kid, maybe five or so, I lived in a nice house and neighborhood in Santa Ana. One of my favorite homes. Come to think of it, this was where I had felt the most stability. I had climbed a high brick wall that surrounded our backyard. I was inching my way to the end of the wall when I slipped. I knew I was going to fall, and somehow, my little hand shot out and barely grabbed the edge of the wall. Then I found the strength to support my whole body weight and pull myself up with my weak little arm. It seemed very strange, and that moment has always stuck with me. It felt as if something had held me because my arm just wasn't strong enough to pull my weight.

That protection never seemed to leave me.

When I was thirteen years old, I lived in North Salt Lake City, Utah. We had just moved from a little apartment about a mile away. Living at the apartment was the most united our family had ever been. My parents worked hard at making a better life for my three sisters, my one brother, and me.

COMFORTABLY INSANE

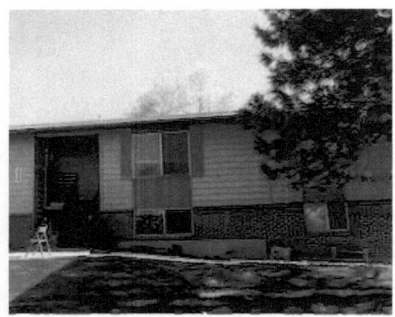

Apartment building where we lived.

During that time, one very happy memory I have is coming home from school one day and finding a makeshift table in the kitchen that consisted of a box covered with a tablecloth. We had just moved there and still did not have furniture. I can still smell the chocolate chip cookies that filled a plate on the table. I can taste the delicious cold milk and how well it went with the cookies. I think that's why I love cookies and milk so much.

I owned my first cool bike here. I loved it! My dad bought it for me at the swap meet. We drove there in his old three-speed Plymouth; the gear changer was by the steering wheel. We had lots of fun in that neighborhood, doing mischievous things like throwing snowballs at cars and through windows. I now realize how dangerous those things were and how easily someone could have gotten hurt. Luckily, no one ever did.

During the summer days, my siblings and I played for endless hours with our friends. We enjoyed riding to the top of the hill where there was a roundabout inwards from the main road. We carefully lined up and said, "On your mark, get set, go!" Then we blasted down the hill as fast as we could. It was exhilarating! I recall wanting to practice and try it on my own one day.

I slowly pedaled up the hill, got to the roundabout, and prepared myself for takeoff. It all started well; I felt like I was flying. I quickly ran into trouble when my chain came off. Since my bike worked as a backpedal brake, I couldn't stop! Exhilaration turned to panic quite quickly as I zoomed down the hill. As I flew down the street, I knew I needed to find a safe place to crash, so I steered

THE BEGINNING

toward the last apartment building and entered the parking lot. I saw a fence and instinctively rode toward it and BAM! I almost blasted right through, but some heavy two-by-fours stopped me. My front wheel came off the frame of the bike, and I splattered on the gravel.

Once I realized I wasn't dead, I checked my body for any broken bones or injuries. Fortunately, there were only two nasty skin burns on my knees. After all these years, if I look closely, I can still locate the scars. I slowly and painfully picked up the pieces, my front wheel in one hand and the frame in the other, and made my way up to my apartment building. I

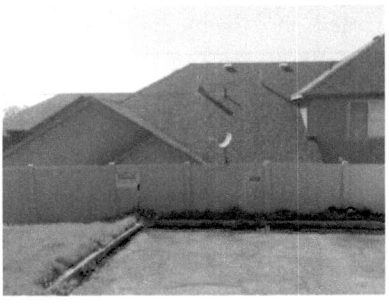

Fence where bike crash happened. Replaced with different material and background house was not there.

was very shaken on the outside; however, on the inside, I felt emotionless. This was the first time I felt disassociated from the reality around me. Soon, this feeling would become almost second nature. I did, however, acknowledge that something had protected me. What it was, I didn't know, but I was definitely protected. I could feel it.

Years earlier when we lived in El Salvador, my mom owned and operated a Montessori school in the city of Santa Ana. We lived in the school; however, my dad lived in San Salvador. I hardly ever saw him. One time, a man showed up at the door, and I ran to tell my mom there was a guy at the door. It turned out to be my dad, so that's how little interaction we had at the time. My mom did her best and was a pillar in keeping things together.

COMFORTABLY INSANE

As I grew older, things slowly changed with my dad. It seemed that with each move, we sometimes grew closer and sometimes grew apart.

One episode as a kid my dad had come home drunk, which was extremely rare. I suspect it wasn't rare that he drank, but he rarely came home drunk. You see, that was a no-no in our family. We, as a family, never drank at home and didn't keep any alcohol there. If we had vices, we did not bring them into the home.

The next thing I knew, I heard him walk out of the house and get into the car. I don't know what came over me, but I instinctively ran outside just in time as he was pulling out. He hit some toys lying around and was in no condition to drive. I ran to the side of the car, and as he stopped, I screamed, "Dad, don't go!" He raised his head and barely focused on me. He turned the car off, came back into the house, and went to bed.

That was a time I felt that weird protection empowering me as well. Perhaps he felt it too. I learned that although he was absent for many years, he always provided for us. Gradually I saw my dad transform his life.

About two years later, we moved into a house that was quite a nice upgrade from the apartment. It had five bedrooms total, including two rooms in the basement. This meant each kid had their own room. There was also a nice front yard with lots of healthy green grass, and the backyard had apricot, apple, and cherry trees, as well as grapevines.

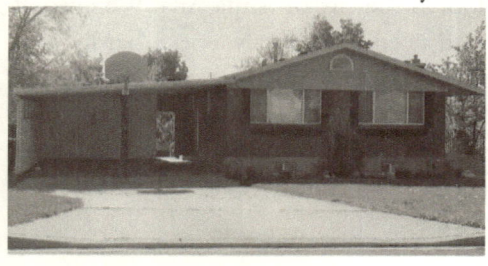
New house where we moved to.

This was a weird time for me because we had been in the new house for about a year when

THE BEGINNING

my mom, two of my siblings, and I had moved to El Salvador once again, and when we returned a couple of years later, I felt confused, and I could feel I had lost the connection to this place.

Since I always felt out of place during my school years in the US, I didn't have many friends, and I pretty much kept to myself to disguise the fact that I didn't fit in. It was something that, to this day, is hard to explain. Though I'm sure there was a component of low self-esteem, I don't think that was entirely it. Just overall relating and feeling like I belonged was impossible for me.

Even though I was experiencing these feelings, seventh grade was a good one for me. I was a great student and pretty much kept up good grades. The change happened in eighth grade. I started to make poor decisions in my attempts to fit in. I remember trying pot and, quite frankly, not liking it. What really struck a chord was beer, the more the better.

The first time I drank was in SLC. It was an unexpected event. I don't think I realized what it meant to get drunk, so the idea of looking for alcohol was more of a mischievous mindset then a want to get drunk. A friend and I were able to get some beers through someone who bought them at the store for us. After drinking them, I remember not knowing if we were drunk. My parents weren't home, so we borrowed my dad's car for a quick drive. My friend was the only one who could drive. We drove around the block, laughing and giggling while listening to heavy metal. We made it back home without any trouble.

Sleeping over at a friend's house in North Salt Lake City, we found a bottle of Johnnie Walker Red Whiskey. I remember drinking a full pint of that stuff and quickly washing it down with a glass of milk. It felt as if it were burning my stomach! I used to think that was the first time I drank, but really it was the first time I blacked out and truly felt the power of alcohol. I couldn't remember anything, except running out of the apartment without a shirt and making snow angels. I recall feeling like death the next day, but I knew in my heart that I had found my new outlet. Or it had found me. It was something I accepted without hesitation. It scared me, but I figured out later in life that alcohol gave me the opportunity to cope with the awkward, restless feelings that plagued me. I felt out of place.

As I was discovering this, I was sent to El Salvador again. I felt so excited that the feeling was quite intoxicating to be there. Externally, I fit in perfectly. The fact that I had come from the US made me quite popular; however, internally, the truth was much different. The beginning was quite fun. Exciting even. There were lots of cute girls, but I was way too shy to talk to them, even though, on the outside, others couldn't tell. But when I drank, I felt I had a true connection to my peers. They drank, and I had discovered I could drink like a fish. It was perfect. I quickly earned the reputation of a wild boy.

Drinking in El Salvador was different than drinking in the US. Drinking was allowed for minors as long as you had money. There was no need to find anyone to buy beer for you. On the downside, a civil war was going on; as a result, we had many run-ins with police officers and soldiers. As scary as they were, they didn't compare to the run-ins with guerrillas. Many times, I had been shot at or almost beaten up; however, I always escaped unscathed.

Once I learned to drink, I couldn't stop. The blackouts started very early on. Sometimes, it was alarming, and other times, it didn't bother me.

Since one of the bars I drank at was right in front of my house in El Salvador, I could pretty much open the door and walk maybe twenty steps across the street and drink whenever I wanted.

But one time, I was the only one in the group who wanted to drink somewhere else. Since I didn't have a car, I decided to run to the

THE BEGINNING

other bar that was four or five miles away. I had to pass by some alleys and dark places that, quite frankly, were very dangerous. When I was halfway there, a guy came out of the darkness. He said, slurring and barely audibly, "Gimme some money." He was definitely drunker than I was. I fearfully said, "I don't have any." No sooner had I finished saying that when he took a swipe at me with a pocketknife and barely nicked my upper inner arm. As I recovered from the surprise, he took a second swipe. That one barely nicked my stomach. I took off running and what saved me was he couldn't run as fast. As I finally got to the other drinking hole, I slumped over to catch my breath.

I soon saw friends happily drinking and joking. I, on the other hand, drank so much that I vacillated between unconsciousness and consciousness. I learned to describe that state almost like a light flickering on and off, like an electrical short circuit. I remember some things but have no recollection of others whatsoever. This became normal. Once I heard that a blackout is when your brain swells so much that you're on the verge of death. If this is so, then it has to be a miracle that I'm alive. Blackouts became my normal.

That night, I came out of a blackout and found myself in the bed of a truck. I didn't recognize the truck and was alarmed and confused. I jumped out at the first stoplight and ran back to the drinking hole. I can only imagine what my friends and the people watching must have thought. Maybe they thought, *what is this crazy kid doing here?* or *why is he disturbing our happy party time?* or possibly, *this kid is putting on a great show.*

I saw the truck again and tried to hide, but they saw me. When they drove close by, it turned out to be my mom and a lawyer who worked for her. I was caught red-handed and busted. She must have told me angrily to get back in the truck! I pretended to comply; however, as we were driving home, I jumped out again,

COMFORTABLY INSANE

ran back to the drinking hole, and drank a few more beers before they came back. This time, they had to take me by force. It took three people to carry me to the truck while I was kicking and screaming.

I have thought a couple of times that just as something was protecting me throughout my life, something else was definitely trying to hurt me. I say that because if I had to be held down by three people, something must have been giving me strength. I don't remember at all; however, I came out of the blackout crying hysterically in bed with my mom sitting by my side. I can only imagine her pain and fright to see her little boy this way. I put my mom through many huge heartaches. This caused me to feel even worse, and the downward spiral continued for years. I felt so bad that it was just better and easier to drink.

I liked going to video booths to watch VHS movies. It was somewhere I could be alone, unbothered, and not have to talk to anybody. One time, when I came home, my mom asked how school was. I lied and said it was okay. Then she said that was weird because the principal had just called her and said that I hadn't been there the last three days.

When the principal approached me with scissors to cut my hair because it was too long in the back (I had previously been warned that I could not show up to school with long hair), I put up my fists and told him that he should too. I remember thinking of Muhammad Ali. Sting like a bee! He looked at me incredulously and walked away, and the next thing I knew, I was kicked out for good.

By this point, my attitude overall had hardened. I was a serious alcohol abuser. When I look back, I'm always amazed by how quickly it progressed for me. All I wanted to do was drink. I felt myself wanting to isolate more and more, not only from others but

THE BEGINNING

also from myself. Alcohol helped me do that. I rejoiced in the release of pressure I felt when getting drunk. It was like magic. One moment I was plagued with insecurity, self-doubt, and feelings of not belonging, and then as if the magician had done his magic trick "Abracadabra," no more stinky, crappy feelings.

Lesson Learned: It's not a requirement to have a troubled childhood or a traumatic event to become an alcoholic. Sometimes, it seems we're just born that way.

The Betrayal

"There comes a time when silence is betrayal."

—Martin Luther King

My brother wanted to go to military school, but I had no interest in attending, especially since it was so far away. The morning my brother was to go to military school, my mom very nicely asked, "Would you like to come with us to drop your brother off at his new school?" I hesitantly thought, *it's the least I could do*, and said, "Okay."

The drive took a little over an hour. The school was located at the top of a very high hill. I remember the winding road to the top seemed endless. Once we arrived, I saw lots of kids dressed in gray uniforms walking hurriedly to what seemed to be their classes. It seemed very organized. Older people dressed in green military uniforms seemed to be in charge.

My mom asked me to help my brother with his bag, so I grabbed it and curiously walked up the walkway that led to the offices. I sat on some chairs right outside the office as they were helping my brother. While walking up the driveway, I thought, *I'm sure glad I don't have to stay here.* I watched for a while and then thought, *I'd better go before my mom leaves me.*

COMFORTABLY INSANE

As I walked out to find my mom and her driver, a man dressed in a green military uniform yelled at me, "Are you the new recruit?" He looked at me as if I were the strangest thing he had ever seen. He was wearing Ray-Ban sunglasses and a cap and looked pretty scary. Although he frightened me, I chuckled and said in Spanish, "Simon loco," the equivalent of "Whatever, dude." I then walked away and looked back at him just to make sure he wasn't following me. I went down the driveway looking for my mom, but I couldn't find her. I thought, *could they really be gone?* A thought hit me, and I opened up the bag I had carried for my brother. It was filled with my stuff. When the reality sunk in, my heart dropped, and I felt fear. Well, actually, I felt betrayed, although, when I think back to this time, I would've done the same thing to my crazy kid. I feel she was desperately trying to help me. I was completely out of touch with reality. I was going down a very dangerous path where I could do whatever I wanted without any discipline.

Lesson Learned: Just because the addict accuses anyone trying to help them of being a betrayer, it doesn't mean it's true. In fact, most of the time, that person is the one who loves them the most!

The First Night

"Fear: an unpleasant, often strong emotion caused by anticipation or awareness of danger."

—Webster's Dictionary

The man dressed in green turned out to be the lieutenant in charge. While in military school, my instincts kicked in. I quickly disassociated emotion and changed to survival mode. This is how I seemed to adapt in life. I learned to do this in any situation, difficult or not. To this day, I recognize those feelings. I'm not sure how I acquired them. Perhaps it was the constant change from El Salvador and Utah for so many years; however, I suspect that even without this change, I would still have these feelings. It's just something that I carried.

After many years of dealing with these feeling, and in my effort to try to understand why I felt like this, I wrote this phrase that seems to fit: *The reasons and triggers may all be different, but the feeling of isolation, depression, incomprehensible demoralization, and darkness seem to always be the same.*

It was easier not to care. The walls came up, and suddenly, I could deal with whatever was before me.

COMFORTABLY INSANE

We were ordered to get our bags and put them in our dormitory, which consisted of noisy metal bunk beds.

The school consisted of three large buildings nestled together in order on a slanted hill. I'm pretty sure they were apartment buildings modified to be a school. The boarding portion of the school was in the last building and at the top of the hill. The actual classes took place on the second level. Each building had three floors. After getting settled, we came back as quickly as possible to report to the lieutenant. He looked at me and screamed, "You are no longer Neal!" He paused for a brief moment to catch his breath, and then continued. "You are now a mere recruit, a maggot, worse than ants, larva, a *cafre* (low-class peasant)!" I was shaken, but, again, you would not have been able to notice this.

The second order of the day was a buzz cut. He hurriedly and aggressively walked us to the barber. I thought, *what! This can't be.* I was shocked. But I kept my composure. I remembered back in the other school when I had been willing to fight my principal to keep my hair; however, here, I wasn't willing to fight anyone because I had no doubt that I'd get my butt whupped. No sting like a bee here! My defiance suddenly turned into survival mode, the smart thing. My hair was promptly buzzed! Next, we changed into our new uniforms. The rest of the afternoon was a haze; however, the first night was embedded in my mind forever.

For dinner that night, we had sweet hotdogs. I had never tasted such a thing. When I took a bite, it oozed white stuff; it was the worst food I had ever tasted. Yuck! I'm sure that people were making great effort to feed us, but I had never tasted such awful food. To make matters worse, or maybe better, we had to eat in under a minute! It was high stress, high impact all the time. The first night was the beginning of a new regimen.

THE FIRST NIGHT

We were sound asleep when, in the middle of the night, a loud bang on one of the bunk beds caused everyone to jump. We awoke to the entire room filled with smoke and people yelling. Things were going so fast, I couldn't understand what they were saying. At the time, I must have been thirteen or fourteen and had never experienced this. To make matters worse, there was a civil war happening in El Salvador, so as I crawled around, I thought we were going to die. I thought for sure we had been attacked by the guerrilla forces. Luckily we hadn't.

I desperately tried to find the way out. When I got a minute to breathe, I started making out the words being yelled. "Formation at the pavilion! Head count!" I recognized one of the voices as the lieutenant, and the others turned out to be some very motivated angry sergeants. Once we were at the pavilion, it turned into a grueling session of what I learned was called "pelotón de maniobra," something I would become very familiar with. What that meant was an intense session of squats, pushups, sit-ups, as well as lifting logs and a heavy rock nicknamed "Juanita," and running up and down the hill until I felt like throwing up. I think nowadays a fitness coach would call that CrossFit. Kind of cute, I guess. Haha.

The only difference is that instead of a fitness coach, we had a highly motivated angry sergeant who would beat you with a bayonet, a wicked-looking piece of wood, or a bamboo stick if you were slacking. Definitely not my favorite activity, and I don't think they do that in CrossFit.

After all this was done, we were ordered back to sleep. I thought, *I've just entered hell.* That would prove to be correct. This had been the longest day. Just that morning, I had been sleeping in my cozy bed in Santa Ana only worried about when I would drink again and what plans I needed to make it happen. After all, it was the only thing I really wanted to do. I fell asleep at the military school thinking, *how am I going to drink here?*

At four a.m., we jumped up again startled with the same loud bang! It was time for a morning jog! Behind the school were dirt roads and houses much like a neighborhood. On one side, you had what seemed to be wilderness, and on the other side, expensive houses; however, in front of the school, the homes were mansions.

All the students, myself included, hurried down the stairs bumping and pushing each other to try to get to formation first. We lined up in formation and started to run. I quickly learned it was quite dangerous because potholes were everywhere. It was pitch dark and impossible to see our feet or where they were landing. It was crucial to always have a firm footing to avoid twisting your ankles while running. Easier said than done. Again, more hell. This was done while singing military songs. Oddly enough, this running would turn out to save my life later.

Once we arrived from our run, it was shower time. Of course, this was at an extremely fast pace. The motivated, angry sergeants were always screaming at the top of their lungs to help us hurry. As if all that wasn't bad enough, the water was ice cold. Back home in Santa Ana, we didn't have hot water either. So we would boil water and mix it with the cold to make warm water and take a standing shower with a bowl; however, the water here was brutally cold! The rules were one minute to get wet, one minute to get clean, and one minute to rinse off. When there are about thirty kids, this was a hard task, especially when you're not used to it. Of course, with time, we became experts, but for now, it was pure hell. Once this was done, we dressed and ate breakfast, and that was rushed as well.

I will confess: I liked my new uniform, although I would never let anyone know. It made me feel important. Maybe even part of

THE FIRST NIGHT

something. I had worn a uniform before, but never this elaborate with a hat, belt buckles, and nicely polished shoes. Oh, and of course, my brand-new buzz cut. It was a weird feeling; however, after getting dressed, I felt a sense of doom. This sense of doom was familiar to me. It felt as if I had always had it. Almost like a dark cloud that followed me around. It was the weirdest part of my life. Something could be going really well or not, but that impending doom feeling seemed to always be there waiting for me, reminding me of its presence.

I quickly put on the emotionless mask to face the next task.

My life was definitely over!

I had a cap in my hand and was fully dressed in my uniform. I walked into the new classroom right before formation started. It was surreal to be there. The room felt very peaceful. I guess when you compare it to everything that had happened the previous night, it was very peaceful. The entire pavilion where all the formations took place was visible from the windows.

I set my hat on one of the desks and walked toward the window. I looked over and saw some students starting to form their lines, everyone in their respective classes. As far as I could tell, they formed six grades (seventh–twelfth). I was still in eighth, just like in Utah, except this school was very different. I must've stood there for five minutes, taking it all in. It seemed I had been there for an eternity, yet it had only been one afternoon and one night. When I turned around, the hat I had placed on the desk was gone. I was sure I had left it there, but it was nowhere to be found. I thought, *no biggie; I'll find it later.* I went to formation without a hat.

To my terror, I immediately realized that they had uniform inspection. Kids were being inspected for facial hair, ironed shirts and pants, shined shoes, shined belt buckles, firm posture, arms straight and close to the waist, and of course, hats. Students who didn't pass the inspection were being called out to the front of the line for a nice *pelotón de maniobra*. Yup, you guessed it; I was chosen. My instincts kicked in, and I quickly learned to not leave your hat unattended—ever! And not only that, I was determined to get my hat back. In that first day of military school, I learned so much. I kept a low profile, observed who was in charge and how things worked, and adapted.

After that first week of school when I got home, I went straight to my room and slept the whole weekend. I was exhausted. I begged and pleaded to be taken out of military school, but in the end, I lost. It was the right place for me. As much as I disliked it, I knew I was in trouble emotionally. I had no discipline, motivation, or convictions; no anchor. And as much as I disliked the school, I knew it was going to give me that. Deep down, I understood I was in the right place and would be taught good principles.

Military school was intense, and to make it worse, El Salvador was in political turmoil at the time, so the guerrilla forces were a real danger for us; in fact, later, we were advised as we traveled to and from the school not to wear our uniforms or anything that would indicate we were military because guerillas could think we were soldiers and shoot us.

Lesson Learned: Order and discipline are tools to be cherished.

The Good, the Bad, and the Beautiful

"One day, someone will come into your life and love you with the good, the bad, and the beautiful. Will you be ready?"

—Neal Linares

I quickly gained confidence in school even though the classes were difficult: algebra, statistics, Spanish grammar, and many other classes that I just felt I didn't understand. Although I was fluent in Spanish, I had a hard time understanding the teachers. But my instincts were strong. I got good grades, which helped me to move up in rank. This gave me a sense of pride. Not only did I do well in school, I learned how to survive. I quickly learned to have a collection of hats both for formal uniforms and for fatigues. I learned I needed backups of just about all pieces of the uniform. Also, I could sell them to the less fortunate who had lost their hats. After a couple of months, my thoughts shifted from wanting to leave to realizing it wasn't so bad. Although I picked up many bad habits here, the balance would prove that I picked up many more good ones.

As you can imagine, a lot of partying happened at the boarding school. Of course, you had to be an expert to hide it, and I was. I always found a way to drink. On the weekends, when I went home,

COMFORTABLY INSANE

I got together with my friends and drank. At school, I creatively found ways to drink.

This was an interesting time because I was excelling in good things, but I continued the bad things.

Although I had always been a huge drinker, in those days, I was also smoking pot. It wasn't my thing, but I did it anyway. I didn't like it because it made me feel so strange. It would not ease my sense of impending doom like alcohol did. For some reason, I always wanted to try things that I knew were difficult, so I organized a little scheme to be able to buy pot in the middle of the week. Mind you, we were in a boarding school, so we couldn't leave.

The night before, I put a set of civilian clothes in my backpack. At night, when no one was looking, I walked over to the wall leading to the wilderness and threw the backpack over. The next day, right before English class started, with my nice teacher, I told him I had to go to the office, then when the time was right, I jumped over the wall, quickly changed to civilian clothes, and ran as fast as possible to catch the bus, which was about a ten-minute solid run. Singing the military songs helped me to keep the pace up. Ha! There I was using all the tools I had to accomplish my mission. I was proud that I could run that way, a benefit of the endless 4 a.m. and other runs we had to do.

From there, I took the bus to the place where they sold pot, which was very dangerous. I walked in the neighborhood as if it were my house. Once I found a dealer, I got the pot and then took the bus ride back. This took me back to where I needed to run another ten solid minutes. Then I changed into my uniform and was back in time for the formation headcount before lunch, all with polished shoes and a sparkling belt buckle. Oh, and, of course, my hat. This was so exciting to me, and no one ever knew. After that initial run,

THE GOOD, THE BAD, AND THE BEAUTIFUL

I did one other run and took pot orders from people in the school. Everything worked out great, but I decided that was way too risky, so I stopped.

I became good at doing these kinds of things, flying under the radar. I remember the colonel, who was the equivalent to a principal, was very happy with me. He saw I had good grades and that I was going up in rank. I was learning!

As crooked as I was, when it came to school and exams, I never cheated. I wasn't interested in cheating. I wanted to earn my grades, and I did. I was only interested in the other stuff because it made me feel like I was accomplishing something that no one knew or had to know. The first year in military school was an exploration for me. I created a foundation. The second year, I felt more seasoned, realizing what I could and couldn't do without getting caught.

When you're a recruit, you get treated like crap. And that happened to me over and over. Even as a second-year recruit, I still dealt with crap, but not as much. When I went home for the weekends, I lost the crappy feeling but the awkward feelings would flood me, and crazy binge drinking was the perfect solution.

The second year of school, the city had something called the international fair. It was unrelated to the school. I had never been there, and the idea of going with my friends was intoxicatingly attractive. I mean that literally, but I also mean I was excited to go. I drank so much during the day that I passed out on a grassy knoll. I couldn't get up. I kind of remember seeing people walking by, but I, for the most part, was knocked out.

As I was lying there completely passed out, I heard someone say, "Neal, is that you? Are you okay?" I knew who it was, but I couldn't answer. It was one of my schoolmates. This was a private school, and I felt embarrassed that I had been seen in that condition—I must have looked scary and awful. I never knew who he was with, but I've always imagined that perhaps he was with his dad or his mom or maybe his sisters or brothers, and he probably told them that I was his schoolmate.

I think that was a very huge point in my developing feelings of low self-worth. Although I had all these qualities and all these capabilities, I just didn't feel I loved myself. I didn't put myself first, or at least, that's what I thought. It's still confusing to me how that works because as I was trying to put myself first, I completely destroyed myself. I later learned that was called self-sabotage.

Military school continued, along with the political turmoil. I was always aware of the turmoil going on. In fact, the second year, which was in 1985, we were sitting at night in front of the school, by the terrace where you could oversee the city, when we heard massive gunfire. Guerrilla forces dressed as soldiers attacked a popular place called Zona Rosa. It was so close to us that we could hear the gunfire. They ended up killing twelve people: four US marines, two US businessmen, one Guatemalan, one Chilean, and four Salvadorians. It was indeed a scary and dangerous time.

Meanwhile, our crazy sergeants were just that: crazy. They were always coming up with ways to humiliate and scare us. Things like naked beauty pageants where we were the contestants. Piggyback squats with a naked classmate on your back. This was normal, and we were used to it. Of course, these activities were done in the middle of the night. When I think back, it was more like a fraternity initiation gone wild that would never end. But the craziness of military school was not responsible for my crazy behavior. If anything, it helped me to tone down my craziness out of fear of getting punished.

But like I mentioned earlier, it wasn't all bad. I enjoyed being part of the military band. When I lived back in Utah, I played trumpet

THE GOOD, THE BAD, AND THE BEAUTIFUL

in junior high. My brother jokingly thought it would be a good idea to let one of the sergeants know. That was enough for the sergeant, and bam, I was a bandmate. I didn't want to be there at first; however, we ended up doing some cool things. But crazy enough, because of that band, I missed *pelotón de maniobra*, and I was really liking those crazy workouts. I have to admit, I was developing a sense of pride being in the school.

Another great advantage of being in this band was that we got to perform in different places. One time, we were invited to perform at a meeting of the bands. We were the smallest band, but we had perfected our choreography. We ran in a march onto the field in unison; we were disciplined. None of the other bands had done that. We were small, but we outperformed all the other bands, and we actually got first place. This was a shocker to us and to our colonel. When we returned with a medium-sized trophy, I could tell the colonel was surprised and delighted. At the same time, we were so happy to share the news. Although at first he thought we were lying or joking, he was really proud of us. This was an amazing feeling.

We occasionally took field trips. One weekend, I was going to take a trip to Guatemala with the school. After asking my parents, they agreed and paid for the trip. The school bus would pick me up in my hometown because it was on the way. I was to wait for the bus at the tollbooth on the highway. I didn't go because they didn't see me where I was waiting, and I did not see them. I was super disappointed; however, something told me I had been saved. I later heard there was a really strong river right where we were to camp. I immediately thought I would have probably fallen in, especially if there had been drinking. I felt blessed I didn't go.

During the last day of school, October 10, 1986, we were participating in a parade of the schools. It was a long four- to five-hour ordeal. We had successfully finished and were so excited because we were going on a trip to the beach with some of our schoolmates. I was buying orange juice because it was deadly hot and humid outside. In my mind, this wasn't a problem because I knew I would soon be enjoying cold beer, though sometimes, at the beach, there was a lack of cold beer. I didn't mind drinking it warm anyways.

As I was paying, the ground started shaking. I freaked out and ran out of the store as fast as I could, thinking that maybe we were under attack by the guerrillas. I happened to look up just in time to see a building split right in half. That was one of the scariest things I had ever seen. I saw the ground move as if it were a thick blanket with waves of air underneath it. An earthquake. Complete chaos ensued. It was mayhem with people running everywhere. I saw the colonel standing on the corner. He was really scared just as we all were. He had almost fallen into a pit but was saved by a student.

A group of us scrambled and got in our truck and sped back to school. We saw buildings collapsed on top of cars. The cars were crushed under the buildings. I imagined people in some cars. I was afraid to look. People were running and screaming as we drove through traffic lights. One of our friends was a tall blond dude. That wasn't common in El Salvador, so when he would get out to stop cars, they actually stopped so we could pass. Also, we all had our uniforms on, so we might have looked like authorities even though we were a bunch of kids. When we got to the school, at first it seemed normal, but it didn't take long to notice that wasn't the case. A van normally parked at the top of the driveway had toppled over. Once in the building, there were several aftershocks. It is a sobering experience to feel the whole building shaking. It felt as if it could crumble on top of you at any moment. Crazy enough, my thought wasn't, *I better hurry so we can go on the trip.* My thought was, *I need to get drunk!*

THE GOOD, THE BAD, AND THE BEAUTIFUL

I was disappointed when we were told the trip was canceled. And just like that, the school year ended. The earthquake took a huge hit on the country. Personally, this experience is another etching in my mind. As shallow as it may seem, I did benefit from the earthquake. You see, I was struggling with algebra. As a result of the chaos, the school board decided that all schools would pass everyone to the next grade automatically due to the earthquake. I guess it made things easier as some administrative buildings were destroyed. This was very good.

Lesson Learned: Learn to recognize the good amidst what seem the worst changes in life.

The Third Year

"Once I acknowledge that life owes me nothing, I have positioned myself so that I can begin to enjoy everything."

—Craig D. Lounsbrough

Military school was going well. I was a third-year senior and had further advanced in rank; however, I was becoming more and more reckless with my drinking, and things were catching up to me. As I continued down the road of drinking and sloppiness, blacking out was normal. And apparently, I had begun to lash out at people when I was drunk. I'm not sure what that meant. To make matters worse, I had accepted that as a by-product. I didn't fight against it but just simply accepted it. Each time I was going to drink, I felt as if I were getting ready to walk on a tightrope way up high in the sky. And each time, I braced myself and drank anyway! One would think that this is when I would make the right decision and simply decide not to. I mean, think about the choice: drink and blackout and perhaps die, or don't drink and stay in your five senses and live. It always amazed me how easily I chose the former over and over. This to me was insanity. But I was past that ability to stop. I honestly felt I didn't have a choice.

Finally, one day, the colonel found out that I was a drinker and not the picture-perfect student I had painted, or at least that he had

COMFORTABLY INSANE

seen. I was out heavily drinking at the fair with my friends from the school. We had a game going where we stacked the empty cups of beer all the way to the roof. Laughing and joking, we were being way too loud and drawing lots of attention to ourselves. We were wearing our T-shirts with the school logo, which was a terrible idea. Again, more sloppiness; this would have never happened in the first year. Our new English teacher was the daughter of the second colonel in charge. She apparently was there and saw us. The next day she quickly informed the colonel. We were severely punished, and my reputation was tarnished. I could tell the colonel was very disappointed. I, however, disassociated and really didn't care in an unhealthy way.

I had always thought that during my third year, I could finally get payback for my first years of being a new recruit; however, the rules of the school were changing. New recruits were being protected from harassment by older students. What?! This didn't help my plans of getting back for the injustices and mistreatment. Ha! In retrospect, I didn't want to hurt anyone, but rather, I think it was the school culture and maybe even military culture. The recruit is the one who gets initiated.

One incident shaped my new attitude toward the school. A group of us had taken some recruits' hats and other things. We were caught and punished, which was okay, but as punishment, the recruits hit us on the back of the legs with the flat blades of the bayonet. While this was a common punishment, it wasn't common for the recruits to do it. Each of the four recruits was allowed to hit each of us twice. I actually bled. This hadn't happened, not even when I was a recruit. It did something to me. I was disenchanted, and honestly, I was done. I'm very stubborn, and I knew I wouldn't change.

My pranks didn't stop there. Every morning during formation, we heard the national hymn of El Salvador. A group of us thought it

THE THIRD YEAR

would be a good idea to remove the needle from the record player that was in the captain's office. We carefully devised a plan. It seemed like a scene out of a movie. We picked the lock, walked in, and removed the needle. I saw some bottles of vodka, but I knew better than to mess with that. Instead, we took some belts and T-shirts. We slowly crawled backwards, wiping our footprints with a towel so there was no evidence. Sure enough, the next day, no hymn was played from the loudspeakers. It was a mystery. Although I must confess, the whole school sang the hymn with no music, and they sounded pretty darn good!

From this point on, it was a downward spiral. Frankly, I didn't care. As a result, I stopped guarding myself. I drank just about every night. I would sneak out and buy beer from the little surrounding stores. One of the local stores would even let us drink with them at their kitchen table. These stores were all around the dirt roads behind the school. It was basically people trying to make ends meet. We call them "tienditas," small stores where people sell chips, cigarettes, and, of course, beer. On some nights, they had dances. All you had to do was drop ten cents into the hat that went around, and you were allowed to dance the next song. Although I never danced because I was too shy, I would always give the ten cents when the hat came around. I would go and hang out and watch the dancing. I was officially in shutdown mode! I no longer cared. Insanity was beginning to settle in my mind. Although I knew it was not normal or okay to be out drinking every day while in military school, I was doing it over and over again, justifying the unjustifiable as okay and normal.

For some reason, I liked to keep pot in my locker. I didn't like to smoke it, but it gave me a thrill to have it in the locker. Someone had noticed that I had a joint well hidden in the upper crevice of the locker. I used to hide cigarettes there, too. He ratted on me. Unfortunately for that person, I knew who he was. A motivated sergeant picked me out of class, took me to the locker, and

COMFORTABLY INSANE

demanded I open it. He knew right where to search. He screamed at me and hit me with the handle of his bayonet. It was actually quite heavy and knocked me out. The next thing I knew, I was lying on the floor after having passed out. No one was in the room, I was bleeding, and my locker was still open. I slowly got up very stunned and in a daze. I checked, and the joint was gone. I checked for all my other possessions in the locker, and they were all there. My head hurt, and to this day, I have a scar as a small bald spot on the right side of my head from that incident. The dude who told on me would go on to experience mysterious losses from food to hats and personal items. You see, I had learned to pick his locker. He never knew who it was.

Lesson Learned: Even if you've gone through something hard and you feel entitled to a certain treatment, it does not mean that you will receive that treatment that you feel so entitled to. But most importantly, that's okay.

Military School Ends

"Not the fruit of experience, but experience itself, is the end."

—Walter Pater

I walked to the terminal in my hometown carrying my heavy bag with a week's full of uniforms. I boarded the usually packed bus. I had been doing this for three years, so I was quite used to it. Normally, my brother accompanied me, but this time, it was just me. It was the beginning of the year. He was in the US and was going to come a few weeks later. I hurriedly looked for a seat. The bus was an experience all in itself. Everyone rushed the bus trying to get a spot. Sometimes, we stood; sometimes, we clung to the stairs of the bus on the back door. We always got to our destination, whatever it took. As I arrived to the city of San Salvador, I slowly walked up, in the blazing heat, the now very familiar hill that led to the school. All motivation was gone. I met some friends who came from different parts of El Salvador. We decided since no one was around, we would go out and party. We quickly found a nice eatery that doubled as a bar where we could have beer. It didn't take long to get obnoxiously drunk. Somewhere along the line, we had purchased a bottle of vodka to make things more interesting.

COMFORTABLY INSANE

When it came time to go back to school, we ran up the hill while singing military songs, the same ones we sang during our morning runs. Yup, and we were singing at the top of our lungs. The nicer homes were here, so I imagine we woke up a few people. Once we arrived, lo and behold, the colonel was there. He had lost faith in me, although my grades were still good. I think he was there to check up on me. Perhaps someone had told on me again or perhaps the neighbors had called to complain. He ordered security not to allow us back in. Instead, he kept us in solitary confinement for the rest of the night. That was the end; we were being expelled. For me, I was done and told myself I didn't care. I wish I could say the same for the rest of my family. I know I hurt my parents. My brother was expecting to come back to the school. I felt a deep sense of remorse and embarrassment. Since no one was around to pick me up (my parents were in the US), I was in confinement for eighteen hours. They finally located one of my favorite aunts. She showed up around 3:00 p.m. I was sweaty, stinky, and hungover. The kids coming to school early in the morning could see us in the confinement area. All the teachers and just about anybody could see us. I didn't care; however, when my aunt arrived, I was momentarily embarrassed. But that quickly left with the thought of being free of that school. So I didn't care much. I knew it would soon be over. The guard was very compassionate. He asked me to clean up a little as he took me to the bathroom. After I did, we were both escorted to the colonel's office. As we walked in, I saw the vodka bottle sitting there on the corner of the colonel's desk as evidence. It had maybe a quarter still left in it. My thought wasn't, *oh, I'm in trouble now*, but rather, *how did we not finish that!* I had to stop myself from asking if I could finish it before I left.

My aunt was so kind. She was very worried and asked me if I wanted to go to her house. I politely asked if she could just drop me off at the bus terminal. On the ride home, I was thinking I just screwed everything up. I felt guilty, worthless, and just plain demoralized. The things the lieutenant called me when I first came

MILITARY SCHOOL ENDS

to the school—maggot, *cafre*, larva—is how I now felt. But then I decided to get drunk that night, and that was all I needed. I wrapped all those feelings and shoved them way down into the pit of my stomach or wherever they went; however, once I arrived in my little town of Santa Ana, I had a problem. No money. I quickly gathered some pants and shirts. I was comforted by the thought that there were more clothes where that came from! I sold them on the black market. It was amazing what you could sell there. Once I had cash, I ran to the first place I could buy a cold beer, and BAM! That made it all better. I knew I was going to blackout. The tightrope came to mind, and I said, *bring it* . . . at least until I came out of my drunken stupor, and that's when I felt the remorse and guilt rush me like a tidal wave. The anxiety, insecurity, pain, and what I now describe as incomprehensible demoralization were relentless. I now understood how and why people take their lives. The only thing that took this away was another drink. Ahh, yes, insanity was settling in quite nicely!

Lesson Learned: My wish of being free of the military school came true, but it was not the best thing to happen to me. Be careful what you wish for. You just might get it.

Life After Military School

"After you have been incarcerated for so long, whatever story is told in the aftermath is beautiful."

—Rhys Ifans

Oddly enough, I kind of missed military school. However bad it was, I knew deep down that the discipline and structure helped me. At the same time, I had a disconnect from full emotion. This was my normal. Nevertheless, I found myself in my hometown of Santa Ana with full freedom, not really knowing what to do. Well, I knew I was always going to get drunk, but I also realized that I wanted to somehow save my school year.

Saving my school year became important to me. I called my aunt Aida. I knew she was aware of what had happened. In my most respectful voice, I said, "Hi, Aunt Aida. I was wondering if you could help me sign up for a school?" There was a very short pause, and she said in a very calming and soft voice, "Of course I will." I always appreciated how she asked no questions but simply helped. I was very grateful for this because I had no explanations.

The next morning, I heard a knock on the door, and it was her. I was ready to go. We walked because we didn't have a car. First stop was the school I had gotten expelled from for trying to fight the principal. My aunt didn't think they would take me back but thought we should try anyway. At that point, I just turned over all my trust to her. Sure enough, after she stated my case, they promptly said no. Second stop was a huge school I had never wanted to go to. The sheer size of it intimidated me. Luckily, they quickly said no as well. All they needed to hear was that I had been expelled from the military school. Frankly, I can't blame them. After all, kids normally go to military school to shape up. We were out of options it seemed when she said, "I have one last resort." It was a school where all the rejects were accepted as they accepted anyone. We got there, and she again stated my case. To my surprise, they didn't want to accept me either. She pleaded with them and mentioned that I was living with my grandpa. Once they knew who my grandpa was, they said they simply couldn't say no, as much as they wanted to! My grandpa was a local businessman. He owned an appliance and furniture store. He was known for offering reasonable payment terms to the community. This was the first time I had experienced someone giving me acceptance due to my family. It was oddly calming to me. My grandpa would often say, "Build a good reputation, and then you can rely on it. You can basically go to sleep." That's why it was important to have great character, he would say.

Well, now I was in school again. I was eternally grateful for my aunt helping me. She has since passed away, but the help she provided has always stayed with me. In this school, I had a new uniform: no hats, belt buckles, or polished shoes. It was weird to be there after so many years in the military school. I naturally didn't take this school seriously, although I was grateful to go to school. One time, just to be a showoff, I got up in the middle of a class. The professor was smoking. I slowly walked up to him, pulled out a cigarette, and asked the professor for a light. He said, surprised, "Of course." I went back to my seat smoking in class as if nothing had happened.

LIFE AFTER MILITARY SCHOOL

The bathrooms were a gathering place for smoking cigarettes and, way in the back of the bathroom, a place for smoking pot. It really seemed like a chimney. I was shocked that the teachers wouldn't say or do anything. I compared it to what would happen in military school: *pelotón de maniobra*, the rock "Juanita," or, worse, expulsion.

This was another weird time in my life. Somehow, I got myself up and went to school. I guess the military discipline was helping me. My parents weren't around, as they were still in the US, and my grandparents were in Guatemala serving a religious mission, so I had to do things on my own. I liked this autonomy, and I felt responsible in this area. I studied little, but I got things done and passed my classes. On the other hand, the drinking was out of control and continuous.

I remember that there were two maids in the house. I found a picture of me in a glass of alcohol under the bed. This must have been some sort of witchcraft and El Salvadorian suspicion: put a person's picture in a full bottle of liquor, and they will become an alcoholic. I laughed and threw it away. I don't think that this was an influence or the reason why I drank so much. But I did acknowledge the bad intentions behind that act. I realized that some people really were simply bad.

After I had found my picture in alcohol, I didn't trust them. I wasn't scared, just had no trust. They always seemed to serve me the weirdest foods, and I would get this eerie feeling that they were watching me from the kitchen as I ate. I recall one time in particular being served some type of black soup. I noticed that they were lingering in the kitchen and made me really uncomfortable. I ate it just because I was hungry and hungover. It didn't take long before I threw up. As I saw the contents coming out of me, I was sure that they were doing something to the food. I never questioned them; I just simply stopped eating at the house. Ha, problem solved.

COMFORTABLY INSANE

I made it through school and got passing grades to save the year. Really, I don't know how that happened, but it did. My days in El Salvador were numbered. I continued to drink heavily. Every weekend was an adventure, sometimes being shot at or getting in fights. These were common occurrences. I truly feel I was protected. Somehow, I survived, thanks, I believe, to a higher power because I just have no other explanations.

> **Lesson Learned:** Sometimes you can accomplish good things just by inertia. Even if you don't mean to, your inner self has the potential to accomplish it.

The Incident

"Trauma is a fact of life. It does not, however, have to be a life sentence."

—Peter A. Levine

This part has been hard to write, and soon you will know why. During this time after military school, I found myself with so much freedom. A friend called me one day and said, "Hey, Neal, let's go to San Salvador. I know some girls who want to meet us." I was excited and said yes. We got on a bus and left for an overnight trip. We drank on the way there. When we got there, we were pretty drunk. Some dudes picked us up at the bus stop. I thought it was odd, but I went with it. At that point, I was more interested in drinking. We arrived at a home where there were only dudes. I asked my friend, "Where are the girls?" He ignored me, which made me very suspicious. I thought he knew the girls we were supposed to meet. So I wondered why he would put us in this situation. Long story short: I was sexually abused. I felt trapped and scared. I recall my friend waking me up at four a.m. or so and nervously saying, "Let's get out of here," which was a surprise.

He seemed to know these people, yet he wanted to get out of there fast as well. I was thrilled about the idea. I wanted to leave. The house was dark. Everything was hazy. My heart, my soul, my whole being was heavy. It felt as if I had entered another level of shame. We looked around and moved very quietly, trying to find some money so we could leave. Finally we found some dude's pants and found a wallet; we took all the money and ran. The sun wasn't even up. I felt dirtier and more broken than I had ever felt in my life. When I finally made it home, I sat in my room. Anger filled my heart. I blamed everyone for my situation and what had happened. I kept this incident to myself and shoved it deep down into the well of emotions.

Lesson Learned: Freedom and crappy decisions can cause a domino effect of bad outcomes.

Back in the USA!

"Land of the free and the home of the brave!"

—The Star Spangled Banner

This time, I was going to do better in Utah. I was determined. I had come back the summer right before eleventh grade. The plan was for me to go to the local high school, Woods Cross, in the fall.

As soon as I arrived to Utah, I immediately started causing trouble. Mike, one of my friends from childhood, came over. He was so excited that I was back. He rode his bike to my house and asked me to join him on a bike ride. I honestly was happy to see him, but I said, "I can't go out," and I never talked to him again. Not sure why I reacted this way. The awkward feelings I had always felt inside were amplified. But now, I also felt dirty. I really didn't want to share time with anyone. I thought I was secure in who I was, but I couldn't get past those feelings.

A month or two into summer, I was hanging out with another school friend. Unlike Mike, he was a drinker. This let me feel okay. I guess I needed to be around people that drank. We drank a lot of beer that day and were playing basketball at the elementary school I had attended when I was smaller. It was near the apartments where I used to live. I had gotten so drunk I could barely stand, but I continued playing. I shot the ball and fell flat on my face. I severely scratched the top of my forehead, nose, and lip. It wasn't a pretty sight.

Later that day, I was driving to another friend's house, and a cop pulled me over. I was so drunk that I could barely stand. The cop took me in. My dad picked me up later. When I went to court, I tried to blame the injuries on him. But the judge knew better and so did my parents. The next day, I woke up with that familiar hangover, both moral and physical. To drown out that moral hangover and my emotions, I had developed a technique that allowed me to drink in my room without anyone finding out. I'd throw the beer cans out my window; however, it was only possible during the winter because the snow would hide the cans. When summer came, I was horrified at the number of beer cans that had piled up. I quickly picked them up before anyone found out. Minor nuances.

Later that day, I got a call from two of my friends to go hang out in downtown Salt Lake City. We met at the bus stop. I was sporting my huge scrapes on my forehead and upper lip. I had put a hat on to try to cover them up but couldn't do that so well because the hat lined up right with my scrape, and it hurt too much. As we waited, my mind was racing. I felt deep anxiety. I didn't want to go, yet I didn't want to stay home. As I was going through this, my mom passed by with my aunt and twin cousin. I love them both! They stopped the car and made me get in. I happily complied. I was embarrassed with my friends and my family but it was the perfect cover so I did not have to explain to my friends that I did not want to go. I often wonder about the coincidence of them showing up at that moment.

Not that I was always protected from my bad choices, but I often found a way to avoid consequences. My older friend Oscar had a car, so it was really convenient to hang out with him. We had

BACK IN THE USA!

decided to go to a club in Salt Lake City. As we drove on State Street a little past 12 a.m., he made a wrong turn onto a one-way street. He immediately tried to correct, but it was too late. The police lights glared at us from behind. The cop walked over to us slowly, pointing a flashlight at us. He was very serious and cautious. He asked us to step out of the car. It did not take long to see how intoxicated we were. He immediately put Oscar in handcuffs and in his police car. He looked at me and must have noticed that I was underage, so he said, "Scram before I arrest you too." He got in the car and left!

So there I was on State Street, not knowing my way around and drunk! I anxiously started to walk home to the best of my ability. At a distance, I saw the State Capitol and realized I needed to go that direction to get to North Salt Lake City. Unfortunately, it also meant walking on the freeway. It was crucial that cars didn't see me, especially a police officer, as I was violating curfew. I walked and walked. It was pitch dark and scary. When I saw car lights, I would find the most convenient bush, cement block, or whatever else I could find to hide behind. As I approached the freeway, there were no more bushes, just the freeway. Thankfully, there were plenty of side railings that I could hide behind as soon as I saw lights. I combined running with walking, and if I saw lights, I would jump to the other side of the cement railing. I would lie still until the car passed, protected by the darkness. That thought was crazy. I had always correlated darkness with insanity, but for now, it was my comfort and protection. I would later understand this better.

This strategy got me to North Salt Lake. Once there, I had to be extra careful because the officers there not only knew me, but they also seemed to always be waiting for me. At least, that's what it felt like. My dad had shared with me that they would wait for him as well. I crouched behind some bushes before entering, carefully scoping out the exit ramp. Military school training was really paying off. Haha. Once I was in the neighborhood, I ran from bush to bush. I knew if I could get to the elementary school, I was home free. That was my turf, and I couldn't get caught there. I knew all the places to hide, so I did just that. I walked past the basketball court where I had fallen and scraped my forehead and upper lip, then went through the small walkway through the chain-link fence right past the school. That's where we played with all our friends as little kids. I thought, *what has happened to me? What am I doing?*

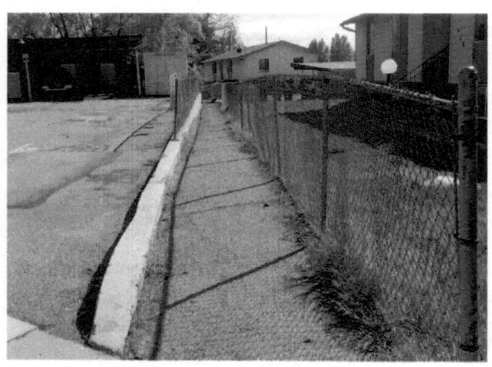

Chained linked fence pathway that connected school and apartment neighborhood.

I ran up the hill past the spot where I had crashed my bike just a few years before. It reminded me of the first time I felt that void of emotion when I had walked with my scraped knees and my dismembered bike. It seemed like an eternity ago. I also ran past my old apartment. I smelled the chocolate chip cookies my mom had made for us when we got home from school that time. I saw another car light come up and instinctively hid behind a bush. Finally, I made it home. I felt safe, but I had no victorious feelings! No victory lap, no sense of accomplishment or relief. Void of emotion, I walked to my room, put the music on as loud as I could without waking anyone, and went to sleep.

By now, I had earned a DUI and a couple of arrests under my belt. My life was simplified. I couldn't drive but I could still drink. Perfect; just the way I liked it!

BACK IN THE USA!

That fall, I started school back up. In military school, I had developed a sense of discipline, but at Woods Cross High School, I had none; however, I was smarter. Why get in trouble with teachers and principals? My old principal from junior high was now in Woods Cross and was very kind to me. He acknowledged once how sharp I looked. It was the weirdest feeling. I dressed much better than the black T-shirts and worn out jeans I used to wear. But inside, I felt so unworthy of everything. The anxious feelings came back strong as ever. They haunted me for many years. I was uneasy and anxious all the time. At nights, I would put music on as loud as I could just to help quiet my mind.

Life continued, as did the arrests. It seemed I was in court every Monday or so. One time, after drinking with my brother and a friend, we ended up at a gas station close to the house. As kids, we stopped here a lot to buy candy and stuff. My brother and friend had gone inside and were playing video games. I was passed out in the car, and when I woke up, I was confused and tried to start the car so I could go home. But I couldn't start it, and the car rolled backwards into the street. Officers promptly came. Once again, they took me in. This time, my dad picked me up. He didn't say a word. He rarely did. He would show his feelings by not saying anything. I was used to it. I was taken to court once again, and the judge suggested strongly I go to a rehab center.

> **Lesson Learned:** Planning to do better is not enough. We need to create solutions through the help of others. Lastly, take action to make sure not everything is wasted.

The First Step

"The first step is always the hardest."

—Unknown

My mom drove me to the rehab center. I had tried everything in my power to manipulate the situation and get out of it. I had no success, so I relied on the skills of bending and adjusting. Good old survival mode. Show no emotion. My mind was the strongest thing I possessed, even though it was insane. Because they wanted me to go, I had to go, but I decided I would just play along until I saw a crack in the system and then jump through to get away and do what I wanted. So, ha! Another learned skill in military school.

Once we got there, my mask came on. A guy who seemed not to have a worry in the world nonchalantly escorted me into a room. He asked me to change into a robe that was lying on the bed. The room was cold and very bright. He also gave me a pamphlet and said, "Write down why you can't stop eating." I thought, *this is one weird request*; however, I quickly figured out they had mistaken me for someone else. I thought, *perfect!* It was the beginnings of the crack I was looking for. I wrote nonsense like I liked eating burgers because they're really tasty and Snickers bars because they're crunchy. Just silly stuff like that. When he came back, he took the writing pad, read it, briefly looked at me, and left. He came back without a word, smile, or any emotion and had me dress back into my clothes. Then he patiently took me to a group of kids who were sitting around in a circle. I felt above everyone in there as soon as I heard the subject. They were discussing the Alcoholics Anonymous step one: "We admitted we were powerless over alcohol—that our lives had become unmanageable."

I was floored and felt sorry for everyone in there. I heard the kids describe how they had suffered with alcohol. One kid had just reached something like thirty days of sobriety, and they asked him to share. He said he felt uncomfortable since I was new. I immediately and energetically offered to leave, but he said no and shared. I was so impressed by the openness of everyone, but not in a good way. I felt sorry for them and wanted to get out of there! After a few hours, I realized I was going to be there for quite some time, maybe a few weeks. I didn't like the idea, but my mindset was strong, and I could go through anything without really showing who I was. I later learned that was easy for me because I had no clue who I was. As I was preparing my mind to get through rehab, surprisingly, my mom came back to get me. She later explained that she talked to her sister, and she had urged her to take me out. Whatever was protecting me had provided the lesson I needed at this moment. All I needed at this moment was to be exposed to step one. I wasn't ready for full rehabilitation, as I needed to first realize I was powerless over alcohol.

Now that I'm a parent, I've begun to understand what turmoil my parents must have gone through in their attempts to help me.

After this experience, I was able to settle down just for a bit in my life. Those kids had an impact on me, and I never forgot what they were saying; I just didn't relate. I ridiculed them whenever I would tell someone about my rehab story. I thought, *I'm not powerless over alcohol. Maybe someday I'll even prove it!*

THE FIRST STEP

It didn't take long to end up with another DUI. It's funny how things tend to work out. I think back and am amazed how easily I got into trouble. This time, my dad was with me in court. The judge said, "I don't ever want to see you here again!" I replied almost mockingly, "Your Honor, I'm going to probably be back next week because I just got caught again this weekend." He threatened to put me in juvenile detention. I laughed a bit and said I would love to go and make some friends there. In reality, inside, I was very afraid. Barely keeping himself from yelling, he said, "I order you to immediately go to juvenile detention." I turned pale; however, my dad intervened. He said, "Your Honor, I'm setting up a business in Miami and leaving in a couple of weeks. Please let me take him with me."

The judge was hesitant at first but agreed to allow that. As we drove home, my dad didn't say a word. But it was understood: I was going to Miami!

> **Lesson Learned:** Some lessons start without us even knowing they have started. We only learn in hindsight as we realize we were being taught a lesson. It's impossible to determine how long it can take to fully learn.

Welcome to Miami

"Yeah, yeah, yeah, yeah, Miami, uh, uh
South beach, bringin' the heat, uh
Ha, ha, can y'all feel that, can y'all feel that?
Jig it out, uh

"Here I am, in the place where I come, to let go
Miami, the base and the sunset low
Everyday like a Mardi Gras, everybody party all day
No work all play, okay

"So we sip a little something, lay the rest the spill
Me an' Charlie at the bar running up a high bill
Nothin' less than ill when we dress to kill
Every time the ladies pass, they be like
(Hi, Will)."

—Will Smith, partial lyrics to "Welcome to Miami"

We loaded the cars. My dad was driving one car, and we were hauling my brother's hatchback Toyota Corolla. My brother had worked so hard at his job to get money to customize it the way he wanted it. He had installed new Pirelli tires and a brand-new pioneer stereo. It had original leather seats and beautiful acrylic blue paint.

Dad and I were going to first drive to Miami to set the groundwork for getting the business up and running and to find a place to live. Then the rest of the family would come. In retrospect, I learned to admire my dad for taking risks. I understood that, sometimes, the decisions he made weren't the best ones, but boy did he fight to provide for his family. And this must have been a huge risk for him. It was a really long trip.

The desire to drink was huge. I slept most of the way as it felt like I couldn't bond with him anyway, but some seeds were planted, eventually improving our father-son relationship. When we arrived to Miami, we immediately got lost and ended up in a bad part of town, hauling a sparkling blue car in the back. We knew we were attracting the wrong attention, so we were relieved when we found our way and arrived at our location, my dad's friend's house where we stayed for about a week. Eventually we found a little apartment on a popular street in Miami called "Calle Ocho." I helped my dad find the building for the new business. We were both excited about this business dream.

Things were very different than SLC. It seemed more like El Salvador but modern. I went from a high school senior class of three hundred students to a senior class of nine hundred. I was in awe of the size of the school. The halls had so many kids you could barely walk. While I was intimidated, you would never know it. I kept to myself and just tried to learn this new environment. At this time, I was fluent in Spanish, but when I listened to most people, I couldn't understand the Spanish they spoke because it was so fast. I was continually asking them to speak English instead. This went on for about a month. It wasn't easy.

WELCOME TO MIAMI

In one of my classes, a dude was flicking papers up front and hit a really big kid. The kid stood up slowly, walked toward him, and just punched him square in the face, then returned to his seat as if nothing happened. I asked the guy if he was okay. He was stunned and then said, "Yeah, I'm fine." I thought, *I'm definitely not in Utah anymore.*

This kid and I became good friends. He asked if I drank, and I enthusiastically said yes!

Here, I would drive my brother's car. One time, during lunch with my newfound friend, we bought a six-pack of beer. I was surprised that there was no issue buying beer, as we were underage. Again, another perk of the Miami lifestyle. We parked at the side of the school's baseball field, which seemed pretty isolated. I opened the beer almost reverently and guzzled it down in one swallow. It was so soothing to me. I know it had been exactly one month since my last drink because I was counting the days. Ever since I had arrived to Miami, I had been with my dad the whole time, so I had not found any way to drink.

While drinking, some police officers saw us. They aggressively pulled up in front of us and asked us to get out of the car. Searching it, they promptly found the three beers that were left. They just opened all three beers and poured them out in the back seat. I knew at that point they weren't going to arrest us, but their style was way different than the officers from Utah. I had a multi-colored stick in the back of the car that had been left there by my mom. She was a schoolteacher and used it to teach kids how to count. The officers thought it was a weapon to fight with, which I thought was very odd. Later, when I learned more about Miami, it all made sense. They had huge problems with gangs, and I was in a rough high school, so every little thing was looked upon as dangerous. I guess beer wasn't so dangerous because they were dealing with cocaine, guns, gangs, and other things. They laughed at us and my beer-smelling car, courtesy of them, and told us to scram!

Believe it or not, I was an exceptional student at Miami Senior High. I had not made many friends and wasn't drinking heavily and was barely going out. Really I was being closely watched by my dad, so it was almost impossible. So I studied and paid attention. I even made the honor roll. Internally, however, I was at an all-time low. I felt out of place—wanting to belong but really not knowing how. Now that I wasn't drinking so much, the feelings of not fitting in returned. I reverted to isolation. I did that very well. About three months in, I started to adjust and began skipping school and partying more and more.

Since my dad had become busy with work, I got more space and freedom. He was unaware that I had now slipped back into bad habits; oddly enough, in spite of this, it felt as if my relationship with my dad improved. I really loved him; I just didn't know how to show it. Truth be told, I think he didn't know how to show it either.

At school, I made a new friend who was a bartender and knew how to make all the drinks, which was great, but I really just liked beer. One Friday night, I was out and about and thought it might be better for me to stay the night at my friend's house because there was going to be lots of drinking. I called my dad to ask permission to sleep over. After a brief silence, he said, "Will you promise not to drive?" I promised. For my dad, your word was really important. He wanted to believe and trust, and he did. In my defense, so did I. I believed that I would be good when I talked to him. But I was fighting a battle that had already been lost; I just didn't realize it. We hung up. I was free. So I started drinking recklessly. I drank and drank. I was surprised how high my tolerance was. In the wee hours, my friends were falling asleep. I, on the other hand, kept

WELCOME TO MIAMI

drinking all through the night. I built a pyramid with the beer cans. I didn't sleep at all and drank by myself.

Early in the morning, when my friends awoke, we decided to go to Miami Beach. The combined IQ level of our group was very low. That became apparent when it was decided I would drive. Well, maybe I decided. When we arrived, I started to experience the flickering lightbulb blackouts, off and on. I ran stop signs and was just being belligerent. This culminated in a multiple car crash. After the crash, I must have been knocked out. I awoke to people screaming. My head was warm with blood coming from a gash above my eye. I got out of the car and saw a guy standing there. I remember him asking if I was okay.

Again I must have blacked out because when I came to, I was in the ER and two officers were asking if I had a license. I said, "Yes, it's in the car." I had no idea what had happened. I was afraid and was alone. It was one of the scariest feelings. I felt that I could die, and no one would care. Apparently, five cars had been involved in the accident. I ran a stop light and a car slammed into me, driven by an older lady. She suffered a broken leg. God was powerful here because no one else died or got hurt. I received stitches on my eye and my leg, and half of my head felt numb. That numbness has never left to this day. I had that familiar feeling of protection with me, except, this time, the guilt was so deep it was hard to feel good about having this type of protection. I truly wanted to disappear or just die.

After this event, things changed in my heart. For the first time, I had deep introspection about my drinking and contemplated rehab. I questioned whether I was powerless to alcohol and if my life had become unmanageable. The next couple of years I thought this over and over. The huge black eye and the stitches all over my body were tangible reminders that I was facing consequences that were beyond my understanding. Nothing made sense.

COMFORTABLY INSANE

My dad picked me up from the hospital. When we arrived home, I sat at the kitchen table. He put both his hands on my shoulders and inspected my eye. I could see his eyes were moist. He then looked me straight in the eyes for a few seconds as if searching for words to say. I also looked back at him, feeling lost and afraid. He then hugged me and held me. Although I couldn't return the hug, I could feel his love. I understood what he was trying to say. I loved him dearly as well.

I went to court several times. A public defender was helping me. Once in court, the lady who had broken her leg chastised me. I was embarrassed and ashamed, but even though no one knew this, I was more grateful that she was okay. After several times of court proceedings, the judge finally said I was guilty. I was then placed on fifty hours of community service, required to attend an alcohol education program with ten classes, and required to pay a fine. I attended the classes very begrudgingly, but I knew I had to be there. I submitted and declared myself a full-blown alcoholic. But I wasn't powerless over it. I know this doesn't make sense, but that's how I felt. It was full insanity. And I liked it!

Actually, the insanity had set in a long time ago for me, but now it was taking over. It was flexing its muscles. I could feel it but couldn't explain it.

I participated in the alcohol education classes and gave as much input as possible. For the community service portion, the guy flat out asked me if I would rather pay him $100, and he would sign off on all the hours. I said yes and somehow got the money together.

As this was winding down, we moved to a slightly better part of town. That meant another school. So this would be my third high school during my senior year. I had started off at Woods Cross High School, then went to Miami High, and ended up at Sunset Senior high. That was a winning formula for chaos.

WELCOME TO MIAMI

I was yearning for something but didn't know what it was or how to explain it. All I knew is that when I drank, the feeling stopped. At Sunset High School, I chose to be very low key. I scraped by to graduation. I made zero friends, and, honestly, the feeling of not belonging was as strong as ever. I became completely detached. I truly felt I was by myself, even though, by this time, my family had all come from Utah, and we were all together.

I still didn't date much. I felt too inadequate.

Lesson Learned: A geographical change doesn't mean things will get better.

The 180

"A man who wants to lead the orchestra must turn his back on the crowd."

—Unknown

I had a thought! I could work and go to El Salvador to see my old friends. Just the mere thought was exhilarating. I could drink freely!

I got a little job at a photography studio to make this trip happen over spring break. Obsession took over in planning this trip. Once in El Salvador, I immediately drove to the beach. I spent lots of time on my own, although I made half-hearted attempts to connect with friends. I went back to Santa Ana to see my grandparents for a bit. Then I returned to the beach to finally connect with friends. The tightrope came to mind. But it didn't stop me.

As I was walking out of the house, I looked back. It was a big house. In the middle, it had an open court with lots of little trees and plants. I could see my grandma sewing on her machine through the plants at the other end of the court. My grandpa was taking a nap. The house was very quiet. I thought, *is that what peace and serenity looks like?* As I started driving and was almost out of the city, I stopped and thought, *why don't you take your grandparents to the beach?* My friends could wait. I did a hurried 180, almost screeching the tires. I barged into the house and excitedly asked if they would like to go have lunch at the beach. My grandma almost jumped out of her chair and immediately said yes, and my grandpa followed. They were so excited and happy. To my surprise, so was I!

All three of us jumped in the car and drove. This was, to this day, one of the most genuinely enjoyable times I have ever had. For me, it was all about them. Not about me. I didn't have to think about me. What a relief! My grandpa told me story after story, and he asked me lots of questions as my grandma chimed in from time to time. I don't remember what they said, but I remember feeling so happy to be with them. We got to the beach, and although I didn't have a camera, the pictures are ingrained in my mind. We arrived at a little restaurant overlooking the ocean. It was beautiful! My grandma wanted fish, so I ordered her a huge whole fish served with a delicious salad. I couldn't believe how big it was. She almost looked small compared to the fish. My grandpa also wanted fish but not as much, so I told them to give him a little fish. I got the same as my grandma. We enjoyed the ocean breeze and talked some more. It was beautiful. We had so much fun; I couldn't hide my smile. I felt connected!

After our meal, we went to a nearby swimming pool. My grandma got in and just enjoyed being in the water; grandpa not so much. He just watched and smiled. I'm not sure what this meant to them, but to me, it was so memorable. Years later, my grandma passed away in Miami. I was so busy partying that I didn't see her much. That gave me a deep sense of guilt that I overcame by this one time that I took my grandparents to the beach.

Later, after dropping them off, I went back to the beach to meet up with my friends and engage in the same old drinking routine.

THE 180

Back in Miami, I fully accepted I was an alcoholic, and honestly, it didn't seem to bother me. Sometimes, I would say to myself, "If I'm an alcoholic, then I want to be the best possible alcoholic." I was more careful, however. Even deeper down inside, I was horrified about the car crash, my lack of memory, and how close I came to hurting and killing people.

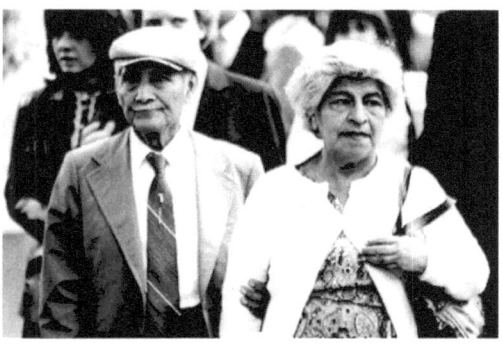

My grandparents at a church function.

During this time, I noticed that the business was really needing me, and I felt I could learn so much. My dad was a very hard worker, and I felt it was a great opportunity. One negative was that working for him meant no pay, at least in the beginning. So I developed a one-two punch: work for him and keep my part-time photography studio job. Also, I sold china, pots, and pans door to door for a while. I saved money and traveled to El Salvador as often as I could. These trips were very unfulfilling to me and full of drunkenness and darkness. While I could feel I needed to stop, as death was close by, I was desperately seeking a connection.

My drinking had become a burden. I always had to get drunk to have fun. If I blacked out, that meant I really partied! Then one day, I started dating this great girl, Janet. I could feel she was special, and I didn't want to mess things up. So, just like that, I stopped. I diverted all my energy into working for my dad and church, and of course, Janet, a full 180.

COMFORTABLY INSANE

Lesson Learned: Listen to the voice of needed change, even if you don't understand. Take action.

PART 2

THE COMFORT OF INSANITY

Eight Years of White Knuckling

"The truth is incontrovertible. Malice may attack it, ignorance may deride it, but in the end, there it is."

—Winston Churchill

You know how you sometimes think you don't have a problem or refuse to admit it? For example, you have a headache, but you don't admit it because you don't want to take an aspirin.

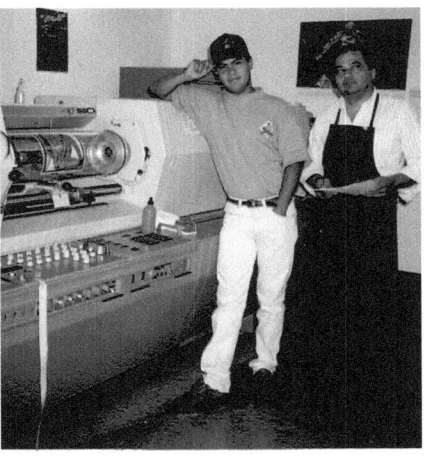

Dad and I. In recently opened business.

Well, that's how this period of time was for me. I became a professional pretender. Part of the reason I had moved to Miami was to work. And a couple of months in, when I almost killed myself and others through the car accident, I realized I could do so much more with my life. Obsession always worked well with me. Now my obsession was to do more with my life and be better. More and more, I worked side

COMFORTABLY INSANE

by side with my dad, although I didn't get paid. I had my other little jobs for money. Once he sent me to deposit a huge check, and I was amazed at this responsibility. Right then and there, I decided I would work for him full time and focus 100 percent. It would become my new obsession. While I didn't have much business experience other than just watching and hanging out at my grandpa's business in El Salvador, I did come from a family of entrepreneurs. I had uncles and cousins that all owned and operated their businesses. As a kid, I once bought a cable box from my cousin for ten dollars. Then I turned around and sold it for eighteen dollars. The feeling was awesome. Although my dad's business was quite different from anything I had ever seen, I was determined to learn. We had what was called a color separation house. It was such a long time ago that present-day technology didn't exist. Photoshop wasn't around either, and computers hadn't made their breakthrough yet, much less the internet. So our job was to prepare the films so the printers could burn plates and print magazines, flyers, postcards, and pretty much all kinds of stuff that went on paper. It was high tech. We used a special machine called a scanner. My dad was a master at it.

During this time, I also got involved with church, trying to do everything perfectly correct. As a result, I was called to serve a mission, and I accepted. I was to serve in Tempe, Arizona. It took lots of preparation. My brother was already serving one, and I wanted to be like him and also please my parents. At least that's what I thought. In retrospect, I think it was more like I wanted to try and feel good about myself. You see, although I wasn't drinking, internally I felt as if I were on a race to get away from me, obsessively doing anything that I could to just get away! I knew there was good inside of me, but no matter how hard I worked or how many times I went to church, I just didn't feel good. But nonstop activity soothed me. Really, it didn't matter what it was as long as I was moving. I didn't have to think if I was in action. So I worked long hours, and the rest of the time, I attended church and church activities.

As focused as I was, I couldn't keep up the standards required to go on a mission. I simply wasn't worthy and didn't qualify. This brought more remorse and frustration. It meant that I couldn't be perfect anymore. Inside, I knew I wasn't, but at least I could pretend on the outside. Confused yet? I know I was. It was a living hell. I learned to live with this feeling, even though it was slowly eating away at me.

Even in sobriety, I felt insane. In a nutshell, I was devoid of emotion, not really understanding if I was doing good or not. But just in case, I performed whatever I was doing perfectly—whether or not it was at church or at work. Outwardly, I felt so mature and in control. Inwardly, I felt nothing but confusion, restlessness, and impending doom that I accepted as normal. I never questioned why I still felt just as insane even in sobriety; however, I'm convinced that it was part of the learning process I was going through. As a result, I just pretended to have everything under control and to be happy. I love the song "The Great Pretender" by the Platters and also the version by Queen. It described me, but no one knew.

With my pretense crumbling a bit when the mission fell through, I needed to do something, so I proposed to my then-girlfriend, Janet. She was and is extremely special!

On the outside, our marriage was a happy one. I spent lots of long hours at work and church, desperately trying to find a release for the way I felt. I went from job duty to church duty to house duty, trying to feel real. Once Janet came into my office at work and handed me a piece of paper. I looked at it and it said, "Congratulations! You're going to be a dad!" I could feel the joy through her. I hugged her and wept a little. I was happy but more confused on what to feel. It was not negative; I wanted this baby more than anything. It was just that, deep down inside, I wasn't sure what or how I was supposed to feel. He was a beautiful baby boy. He was born healthy and bright!

Work was starting to pay off financially. Shortly after, we purchased a brand-new home, built to our specs. While I rarely thought about drinking simply because I was busy doing things, I still didn't feel emotion. At work, I occasionally received wine bottles as gifts, either for Christmas or other holidays. I simply dumped them down the drain without even a second thought. I even threw away my good collection of CDs because they didn't fit my religious beliefs. Really, in my mind, I was going to be perfect.

Everything was about business and church. Oddly enough, that was pretty safe. At work, I could hide (even though I didn't realize I was hiding) behind the "I'm so busy" wall. At church, I could hide behind the "I'm so perfect" wall.

This was my life for years, going to work at four in the morning, working all day, sometimes not coming home till the next day, sleeping for a little bit, and then off to work again. That's how it was. This resulted in good things. The business succeeded. Janet seemed to understand that hard work was required and seemed happy, at least for a little bit. Unfortunately for both of us, it was a ticking time bomb. We were just clueless that it was there. Our boy was beautiful. I loved and still love him. I understood that I just didn't know how to show it that well. I desperately wanted to be an example for him. So there were definitely good things happening, and I'm grateful for them.

Yet the familiar feeling of impending doom was still there. Actually, I was learning to recognize it more clearly. I was experiencing severe anxiety, unable to sleep or sit peacefully at home, having recurring nightmares, and unable to make deep connections.

EIGHT YEARS OF WHITE KNUCKLING

I had two years of sobriety before getting married, then three more years during my marriage. I could feel myself bursting at the seams. I was restless, irritable, and discontent. After the sixth year of being sober, I was still keeping it together, but my mind started to wander. We took a super fun trip to Orlando, Florida, with my little sister, my wife, and other friends. We went to Pleasure Island, which had seven nightclubs. No one drank, but we all danced. It felt so comfortable and free because everyone around us was drinking. Even if I wasn't, it was exhilarating. We jumped around from club to club but mostly stayed in the disco club. As we walked, I was transfixed watching people drink and having so much fun. I watched this guy with a huge blue and gold beer can. He took the biggest drink. I was so curious. As the night went on, I saw many people with the same beer cans. The image would live in my mind for the next couple of years.

My subconscious mind had taken good notes. I didn't realize it, but seeds had been planted inside that were beginning to sprout. Most definitely, eight years of white knuckling were taking a toll.

Lesson Learned: Alcoholics and addicts have a tremendous amount of misdirected willpower.

I Feared Sanity

"This very real feeling of inferiority is magnified by his childish sensitivity and it is this state of affairs which generates in him that insatiable, abnormal craving for self-approval and success in the eyes of the world. Still a child, he cries for the moon. And the moon, it seems, won't have him!"

—*The Language of the Heart*, p. 102

By the seventh year of sobriety, I was barely keeping things together. I needed an out fast, as I could no longer bear my life. Janet was also worried for me. I would continually ask her, "How do you feel? Are you happy?" She was supportive and tried to make me see things in a different way. During this time, my dear cousin Walter, whom I had looked up to almost as a father figure, passed away. I traveled to El Salvador for his funeral. Although it was a sad experience and I was devastated, I fixated on the idea of coming back for a vacation. I returned home, and my anxiety and restlessness turned to continuous depression, a familiar, natural feeling. My comfort zone. Insanity! I announced to Janet, "I'm going to El Salvador for one week by myself!"

Alarmed, she asked, "Why don't we all go?"

"I need to go alone; I need to breathe. I feel like I'm going to suffocate."

COMFORTABLY INSANE

She insisted we could all go. But I was determined, and I wasn't asking for permission.

She took me to the airport. I could tell she was devastated. She didn't know what to do. I was as stubborn as a mule and dead set on leaving. When I look back, this was one of the times when I wish I could have acted differently, taken a step back, and considered how she felt. She didn't deserve to go through this type of pain, especially while carrying our beautiful baby boy in her arms; however, inside, I was dying. I also didn't know what to do and just needed to get away. During the trip, I reconnected with many childhood friends, attended parties, and connected with a female friend. Although nothing happened, seeds were planted. I didn't drink one ounce of alcohol, but I stayed out till late at parties. Looking back, I had no clue the trouble I was in. There was no way of learning this lesson other than going through it. While the thing protecting me—whatever it was—was still there, it wasn't giving me an easy pass. It was starting to teach me things about myself that I simply didn't understand. This trip proved to be the end for our marriage. I had planned to stay an extra three days from the time I bought my tickets; however, I didn't share that with Janet at the time. I, instead, mentioned it when I spoke to her on the phone. She immediately took things the wrong way, accusing me of infidelity. Although I hadn't been unfaithful physically, I had been with my heart. At the time, I was completely offended. After all these years of unwavering work ethic, church attendance, and complete devotion to her and my family, I wasn't granted any benefit of the doubt. This infuriated me. And it was everyone's fault. And how was it possible that she didn't even believe me? Finally, the trip was over, and it was time to come home.

I FEARED SANITY

Lesson Learned: Relapses happen way before the actual relapse.

The Big Burst!

"We were having trouble with personal relationships, we couldn't control our emotional natures, we were a prey to misery and depression, we couldn't make a living, we had a feeling of uselessness, we were full of fear, we were unhappy, we couldn't seem to be of real help to other people."

—*Alcoholics Anonymous*, p. 52

I arrived at Miami international with the feeling of impending doom at an all-time high. I had felt this level of intensity of doom once before when I visited some friends in LA. On that trip, I had drunk so much and was so morally bankrupt, I cried the whole flight home. That's how I felt now. It was odd because I hadn't gotten drunk or cheated. I cried for the two-hour flight, releasing some repressed feelings.

My dad picked me up at the airport. I quickly put on my "I'm perfect" mask. I asked if he could take me home instead of the office. He told me Janet had passed by the office and threw a couple of garbage bags full of my clothes. I was so upset. Internally, I thought, *this is it; I'm getting divorced*. After hearing this, I pivoted and asked my dad if I could stay with them. He said, "No problem; take all the time you need."

COMFORTABLY INSANE

I resettled at my parents' home and avoided talking to my wife as much as possible. An opportunity for a business trip was coming up in Puerto Rico for the launch of a client's magazine. I wanted to go, but more than anything, I just wanted to get away from Miami. I decided that I was going to drink. Once I made that decision, this idea came front and center over every other thought. That was all I could think about night and day. I planned how I was going to do it. I figured I would arrive to Puerto Rico, get settled in the hotel, and then just go to the nearest bar and drink. I thought maybe I could have one of those blue and gold beer cans I had seen a few years ago. The images were so vivid and clear in my mind. After two months or so of obsessively planning my return to drinking, the day finally came.

With my heart beating, I wondered so many things, like what was it going to taste like? Would anyone know I was drinking after eight years? How many would I drink? Would I black out? But oddly enough, my white knuckling fists seemed to be at rest for the first time since I had stopped drinking eight years ago. As intense as these feelings were, at the same time, I was relaxed. The present chaotic feelings were a small price to pay for the peace that would soon come.

> **Lesson Learned:** My addictive substance is my medication to take me away from the real problem, which is myself. And if I am the problem, I am also the solution!

At the Bar

"[L]et us not suppose even for an instant that we are not under constraint . . . Our former tyrant, King Alcohol, always stands ready again to clutch us to him. Therefore, freedom from alcohol is the great 'must' that has to be achieved, else we go mad or die."

—*As Bill Sees It*, p. 134

I was finally there. I carefully sat down and quickly located the server. The bar was well lit, mostly from the natural daylight. While I wanted to order the blue and gold can, I was too shy, worried I would get the name wrong and they would know I was about to drink after eight years. So I just said, "Give me a beer." She asked me what kind, and I pointed at the bottles sitting on the bar. She brought one over and placed it on the table.

I looked at it for about a minute before touching it. Once I grabbed it, I could feel the coldness. A rush of panic and calmness came over me all at the same time. I looked around and saw no one looking at me. I swiftly brought it to my lips and chugged. I drank the whole thing at once. Immediately, I felt a warm sensation as the alcohol flooded my body. I looked for the waitress again and asked for another. By the time I got the second beer, I felt just a tinge of comfort. Anxiety slowly began to recede; however, I could still feel the weight of the world with my current life in Miami. Once I got the second beer, I asked her if she could bring another.

She said, "You're off to a fast start."

I took this as encouragement. I thought, no worries, Neal, oblivion is coming soon!

As soon as she turned around, I brought the second bottle to my lips. This time, I didn't care who was looking. I just chugged. I might have finished that one quicker than the first one. Feeling my body warm up even more, my mind began to relax, and my heart and anxiety soothed. I thought, *one and twenty more*. (In Spanish, "Una y veinte más.") That became my motto. Once she came back with the third bottle, I asked for the check. I drank the third one just as fast as the other two. And bam! I was back. It always amazed me that after eight years of not drinking, it took no more than thirty minutes to be exactly where I was before. By this time, the anxious and impending doom feelings were almost gone. I paid and headed toward a disco club. The road was dark and lonely.

Once I arrived at the dark, smoky disco club, I felt out of place, but no worries; I knew the solution. I quickly ordered more beer. I confess I don't know how much I drank and don't remember how I got back to the hotel.

I woke up at noon (I hadn't slept that late in a long time) to a ringing phone. I didn't answer. With that, I got up, did some pushups and sit-ups, and shadow boxed until I broke a sweat. Working out when I was in military school always seemed to help when I was hungover, so I figured I would try it again. Actually, I was feeling pretty good; however, I could feel the anxiety coming back. Someone knocked at my door. I knew I'd better open it. It was the hotel guest attendant letting me know that my client had been trying to call me. Also, my mom was looking for me. Yup, my

AT THE BAR

mom was always looking for me. It was so out of character for me to be unreachable that I guess I had everyone worried.

Later that night was the magazine launch event. To my delight, it was a full-blown party with an open bar. I indulged and blacked out just as quickly again.

On my way back to Miami, I decided I wouldn't drink. I was worried about getting home, hiding the fact that I had drunk, and working things out with Janet. Sometime after I came home from Puerto Rico, the insidious thought came: *I'm going to drink again!* That's all it took. My mind took over. I scouted different bars, planned how to do it without anyone knowing, and proactively looked for the cracks. My old skills worked as the answers revealed themselves with time. I enjoyed thinking about it. It was an obsession. I thought, *this time I'm really going to get that blue and gold beer.* Although I had felt insane while living in sobriety, this feeling was different. I truly felt that I was going to be happy. Alcoholic insanity, I have missed you!

Sure enough, three months later, the day came, and BAM, I was at the bar again. As I sat down, I saw some huge mugs. I thought, *well, tonight it won't be the canned beer, but I'll take one of those glasses. Those are a little tougher to chug, but no worries; I got this!* I made friends with the bartender very quickly. After three of those, I decided to go home. Janet had gone on a trip, which worked out well because she didn't know I had started drinking. In my mind, I hadn't. This was just a little distraction. I bought some beers, went home, and blacked out. Drinking alone and justifying it as normal. Yup, insanity was back, or the reality was it had never left; it was just manifesting itself in a different form.

In alcoholic terms, I was in more trouble than I knew. I was in a full-blown methodical spread-out relapse.

COMFORTABLY INSANE

Lesson Learned: Alcohol addiction patiently waits to snare you back in its grasp with the same exact power it held over you before.

The Decline

"They are restless, irritable and discontented, unless they can again experience the sense of ease and comfort which comes at once by taking a few drinks—drinks which they see others taking with impunity."

—*"The Doctor's Opinion,"* Alcoholics Anonymous

The decline. That is exactly how I describe the next portion of my life. I wanted freedom, happiness, overall peace, and serenity inside. But my approach to try to get them was a fantasy. A fake. Even a bigger fake than what I had been doing during the eight years of white knuckling. I just didn't know it yet.

A few weeks after declaring I would drink again, I creatively and actively invented situations for me to drink. Nothing seemed impossible. I was back with Janet at the time, but it didn't take long before I was out of the house again and back at my parents' house. In less than a year, we went through a painful divorce, and I left the church. I was offended by some of the leaders. In reality, I was just looking for an excuse. Any excuse would do. They gave it to me; I took it and ran. I later realized that it had nothing to do with them. I was going to leave no matter what.

COMFORTABLY INSANE

At this time, I was going to nightclubs just about every other night. I would wait till my parents were asleep and then carefully walk out of the house. In the mornings, I reeked of alcohol. The only thing that gave me comfort was knowing when I would drink again. I could work for as many hours as necessary, as long as I knew when I was going to drink again. Thus, nightclubs became my safe haven. I felt exhilarated and liberated even though I drank and danced by myself since I didn't have friends.

Again, for me, nothing was real. I was really trying to be alone without being alone. I wasn't a good dancer, but one time I walked into the club having had a few drinks. I don't really remember what happened. But next thing I knew, it was about four in the morning, and I was sitting on a bench with a group of people I had never met before. Apparently, I had engaged in a dance-off with one of the dudes there. I came out of the blackout to a girl saying, "You're a really good dancer." I thought it was funny, but at the same time, I had no clue what she was talking about. This became normal for me.

After two or three years of this type of lonely drinking, I made some friends. We all drank together, but it felt like I drank more than them in a desperate need to try to be normal and happy.

Along with making some friends, I entered several failed relationships during this time. One of these relationships was with a woman named Julie. For the first time, I dated someone who drank and lost control just as much as I did. On two occasions, I ended up in jail for fighting with her. This was the first time besides the DUIs that I had legal trouble.

Together, we were a ticking time bomb; however, we did love each other and talked about the feeling. Julie would say, "Do you ever feel like you're worried about something but don't know what?" Although I never could answer directly, I knew exactly what she

THE DECLINE

meant. We decided once that we might have a problem and would check out an AA meeting.

For the first time ever, we both walked into an AA meeting. The tables and chairs were a bit disorganized; however, it was full of people. At the beginning of the meeting, the guy conducting the meeting said, "Anyone in here who wants to give up the fight and stop drinking for just one day, you can come pick up a white chip." I had no intention of going and getting a chip. I found myself rationalizing and thinking, *it's really not that bad*; however, I was blown away when I saw Julie slowly get up and walk over to get a white chip. It was one of the most courageous things I had ever seen. I was so proud of her; however, for me, I had amnesia of the past!

Although she stopped for a few days and I toned down my drinking as a result of this meeting, this relationship was a turbulent one. We constantly fought. We constantly drank. It was an endless cycle of worry, hurt, and pain. After a fight one time, we never spoke again, and it simply ended.

At a bar, I met Susan, who became my second wife. Ironically, the first time we met, I was so drunk I couldn't put her phone number in my phone. I asked her to please save it in my phone. I called six months later. In a nutshell, this defined this relationship: a drunken stupor.

By this time, I was a regular at the bars. Some bartenders liked me; some didn't. I was a weekend warrior drinking lots, and Susan was a willing participant with me. She was oblivious to how deep in trouble I was. While we had developed some friends, our social scene always took place at the bar. It seemed that everyone could drink like normal people, except me. I was always causing some sort of trouble. Susan was patient for the most part.

COMFORTABLY INSANE

Along with my newfound relationship with Susan, I worked on maintaining a relationship with the son I had with my first wife. While I tried not to let him see me drink and succeeded for the most part, unfortunately, he did see me drunk out of my mind more than once.

Out of all the things that have happened to me up until this point, my biggest regret is not being able to connect more with my beautiful son. He was and still is such a special boy. In fact, this book is dedicated to him, to share with him that change is possible.

It really is the biggest message I can share. It's the same exact message that my dad shared with me. You can change!

Something happened between my son and me that, to this day, I cringe when I think of it. It is not a drastic event, but it embodied so many moments and my inability to take action to improve. My son must have been about ten years old. Susan and I had booked one of the nicer hotels (I got a deal through work) over the weekend in Miami Beach. We called it a mini vacation. My dear boy was so happy. We went to the pool. I got a beer and sat down to watch him play in the pool. He couldn't swim well at the time, and he came to the corner of the pool and looked at me with his eyes pleading with me to come swim with him. While he didn't say the words outright, he continued to look at me for a bit. We made eye contact. I didn't budge. I didn't move. I just sat there. I felt it to my very core. Susan sat by me. I often wonder if she questioned why I didn't go play with my son, or maybe she was just oblivious to the whole situation. That night, I blacked out. I had a bottle of whiskey by the bed and just drank. The next day, we took him home, and I drank some more.

I have never forgotten that night. Of course, it wasn't the only night I had let him down. But it's the one that represented all those years of not being the father that I had wished to be. This is one

THE DECLINE

thing I cannot redo or make right. Why couldn't I have just swam and played with him?

> **Lesson Learned:** The law of gravity, which states that what goes up must come down, applies to alcohol and addiction relapse. Relapse will take you down!

End of Fantasy

*"From covering the truth with lies,
I lied to myself without knowing that I had lost
I always waited to receive when I never offered anything.
Today it's my turn to cry; rather than always laughing,
I forgot to live."*

—Partial lyrics to Julio Iglesias'
"Me Olvidé De Vivir"

My life had become a series of drunken episodes. I was a regular drunk at the bars. Bartenders knew me and sometimes had my beer ready at the bar before I sat down. Some would, every now and then, offer words of concern for me. My binges were no longer restricted to weekends. They had gradually extended to Mondays, Tuesdays, and at times, Wednesdays. I had become an everyday drinker. I marked it as a victory when I was able to stop just before blacking out and be functional the next morning.

On some days, after waking up with a morning hangover, I would sit in the living room until Susan left for work. She was growing impatient. She could drink, but rarely did she lose her senses like I would. I sat, watching black and white movies with the sound off, feeling the full brunt of incomprehensible demoralization. Some Mondays, I went to the bars around nine-thirty or ten in the morning and helped set the ice machine so I could get beers earlier than the normal time. Bartenders thought it was funny. And I always made sure to tip well.

On Tuesdays, I would sit at home when I wasn't able to make it to work and watch silent black and white movies. I had gotten used to watching movies with no sound. The quiet felt calming. I was intrigued by the fact that all the actors were all dead. I don't know what that meant to my mental state. At times, I thought that meant I wanted to die as well. I also liked watching movies with the big bands in black and white. Same mentality. Everyone there was dead. Maybe I thought, *they're all dead, so they can't judge me.* To this day, I have no idea why I preferred watching these movies. They somehow seemed to comfort me.

My drinking got so bad I would drop important responsibilities. For example, one time I had a full weekend planned with my beautiful son. I had a business golf tournament, and the plan was to pick him up and spend the weekend together. Honestly, I had never golfed before and had little interest; however, I knew there was going to be beer, and it was good for business. I arrived at nine in the morning, and my client set the teams. After I had the first sip of beer, it only took a few minutes before I called my son's mom at nine-thirty to cancel the trip. I knew without any doubt that I was going to drink all weekend. Nothing else mattered. When this happened, which was almost always, I would think, *is this going to be the time? Will I die this time?* The tightrope thought would come. But no matter how scary that thought was, I always chose to drink. Alcohol was making me, or had made me, insane. Sometimes I would think, *alcohol is my excuse for being insane. What's yours?*

Approximately ten years after starting to drink again, I had that pivotal moment I mentioned at the start. That morning, Susan had

END OF FANTASY

left a note for me that said, "You need to do something about your drinking, or you need to leave." I brushed it off, not realizing how serious she was.

I knew later that day Susan and I were going to see her brother-in-law perform at a bar. I had decided earlier that day to meet at another bar with one of my buddies to warm up with a few beers, so I left work early.

After an afternoon of drinking and watching Susan's brother-in-law at the club, the cops found me walking uncontrollably on the streets of Miami. Of course, as I mentioned at the start, I was so drunk I thought the red and blue lights of the cop car meant it was Christmas.

They questioned me as I walked. Apparently, I was amusing them as they thought I was funny and liked me. I might have told them what I wanted for Christmas, explaining to them that I thought they were Santa Claus. They were asking if I had crashed my car and wanted to know where my car was. I was flickering in and out of my blackout. I thought, very confused, *yeah where's my car? Maybe I should call the police to help me find it.*

The officers determined I was safe and that I obviously didn't have a car, hadn't been in a crash recently, and wasn't running away from some crime scene. I was just your regular run-of-the-mill drunk. The funny wino. They instructed me to get in the car so they could take me home.

So there we were. I lived in a gated community, and the guards knew me well. And, of course, the fact that I was in a police car caused them to let us right through. I showed them the house. They could not hide their amusement and laughter. I said, "Hey, I don't have my keys, so I'll jump the fence. Can you hang around until I make it over?" They just laughed even more. So I staggered to the fence and jumped over. It was a hard fall to the other side. I was used to it. Many times, I had woken up with a broken phone and camera in my pocket. Bruises on my legs. Cuts on my hands. All mysterious, not knowing what or how it had happened. I raised my hands over the fence and gave them a thumbs-up. They left. I walked to the sliding door in the backyard, and it was locked. I knew Susan was in there and could hear me. At this point, I felt anger. *How could she have left me at the club!* I looked for hidden keys and nothing. I sat for a moment. Then I got an idea. I picked up one of the plants and threw it through the office window and carefully climbed in. When I look back, I don't know how I made it through the window with so little damage to my body. I mean, I cut my hands and arms, but my torso was untouched. Once I was in, I ran to the room, but the door was locked. I somehow picked it open and screamed at her, "How could you leave me!" I managed to scare her, and she tried to run out of the house. At that point, I heard her scream, "I'm calling your dad." Somehow, that calmed me down, and I went to sleep on the couch.

The next thing I knew, my dad was waking me up. It must have been three or four in the morning. I was still drunk but not in short-circuit mode. I said, "Dad, I'm so sorry. I can't believe she called you." I remembered I had a cigarette somewhere hidden in the couch, so I started to look for it.

My dad said, "Come on; let's go. You need to leave the house."

During my first divorce when Janet had kicked me out of the house, I complied with her wishes and then found out later I wasn't allowed to return home. I didn't want to go through that again, so I refused to leave. I sat up and could see her standing in the dark. I was so upset at her. But more than anything, I was remorseful. I was hurting another amazing woman. She had had it, and I couldn't blame her. I could only imagine what was going through her mind; perhaps she thought, *I've given him everything I know how to give, and he's getting worse.* If those were her thoughts, she

END OF FANTASY

was right. It was never going to work; neither of us realized how sick I was. I had managed to put that woman through a living hell. I suspect that when she stood there in the dark, watching my dad plead with me, it was the very moment she gave up on me. But maybe it could have been long before. I ran into the bedroom, shut the door, and went to sleep. I later heard her and my dad talking, and then they started picking the lock. The door opened, she grabbed some things, and she was gone. I told myself I didn't care one bit.

The next day, I woke up to the normal deep and incomprehensible feeling of demoralization. Nothing could take that away but more alcohol. I dragged myself out of bed and managed to get a drink at the closest bar, which was a two-mile walk. I didn't want to drive because I might black out. I drank all day and never heard from her. The darkness that night engulfed me like a hot, suffocating blanket. I had to drink more, so I did at home alone. This was also quite common for me. Although I knew darkness, this level was new. This was black hole darkness. I have seen movies or documentaries of people in an insane asylum. That's the type of darkness I was going through, where nothing makes sense or ever could. This is what people must feel right before they kill themselves.

The next day, I woke up even worse. I had to get out to the bar. I was obsessively looking at my phone, and I might have even called her or texted her. But I got no answer. Or maybe not. I cannot remember. What I do remember was her texting and saying, "I'll be at the house around five this evening to get the rest of my things. Please don't be there."

I felt comforted that she had reached out. I thought, *okay, no worries; I won't be there*. I didn't think of it much and was sure it was just a phase and that we would get back to normal, whatever that was.

COMFORTABLY INSANE

Somehow, the rest of the weekend, I managed to drink like a normal human being, which in my illogical mind meant I did not black out. A twelve-pack of beer before eleven at night. The next day, when I woke up, I was startled and shaking. It was Monday. I knew I had to make it to work even though things had not been normal. When I got to my office, I checked my emails and, sure enough, there was her email, very simple, very to the point. Basically, it said she was filing for divorce, followed by a few instructions on what to expect. I was shattered!

I went home and at the entrance fell over in agony. I was in the fetal position on the floor, crying and saying, "What have I done?" I was so sorry I had ever hurt Susan. But I was sorrier for my life, for my son, and for everyone in my life that I had hurt.

The next few days were a haze. I was going to wait for her. As I did this, I drank more than normal. I was blacking out and confused and didn't know if it was night or day. When I would wake, I would temporarily forget and wonder where she was, only to be reminded.

I thought, *what is Susan going through? She must really be happy without me!* I dubbed myself the monster that no one wanted to be with. Even though this was happening and I did blame myself, I didn't know how to accept responsibility. Little did I know that this was the beginning of another very crucial lesson.

During this time, I went to the bar to feel comfortably insane! I thought how silly everything was. I continually drank myself to a blackout and, the next day, found myself sitting at the bar again. Sometimes, people who knew me would say, "I cannot believe you're back!"

One time, the bar had just opened. As usual, I was the first one there and the last one out. The smell of the bar gave me comfort. The bar was empty, and I put my head down to look at my phone.

END OF FANTASY

As I was looking down, I felt surrounded by people and noise just as if the bar were full. When I pulled my head back up and looked around, it was empty. I was hallucinating and fully aware. That was a new symptom for me. I had never experienced that before, and it really made me paranoid. Also, I began thinking everyone was talking about me. It was a horrible feeling, and the only cure seemed to be more alcohol. I was insanely happy to comply.

I knew this darkness. It felt as if darkness itself was smirking at me and saying, "I got you now." While I was keenly aware that the thing that had been protecting me all these years had given me a second chance, I figured I had screwed that up and taken it for granted. With all these emotions and failures, all I could think about was when would I drink again? The answer came quickly; it would be that same afternoon. My solution was to keep being insane. It really was sooooo comfortable here.

Lesson Learned: The allure of alcohol and addiction was merely an illusion. I looked for happiness and freedom, but it brought destruction and misery.

Stop!

"To get something you never had, you have to do something you never did. When God takes something from your grasp, he's not punishing you, but merely opening your hands to receive something better."

—Unknown

Nothing could have prepared me for the next years of my life. In my mind, I was going to do everything in my power to prevent a second divorce. By this time, I had been actively drinking for ten years; however, it soon became apparent that I didn't have an option. My little sister suggested I read a book called *Divorce Busting* by Michele Weiner-Davis.

I read it cover to cover. I thought, *this is the solution to our marriage. We don't have to get a divorce.* As I read the book, naturally I was drinking. Yup, a little more insanity for you.

I made phone calls to health professionals, lawyers, friends, and family. They counseled me about life and divorce. I knew in my heart, the final solution would be to join AA; well, it was more of a frightening suspicion.

COMFORTABLY INSANE

One time, I met up with some friends I had in common with Susan. We would routinely get together and drink. I could tell they felt awful about the whole thing. They drank with me for a bit, and then they left. I could feel the walls closing in and honestly felt no one wanted anything to do with me. I stayed at the bar and ordered another pitcher of beer. I looked at it and said, "This will be my last pitcher; I quit." I drank it almost by force. I paid and left. I soon found myself at another bar with another pitcher. I thought, *this thing has such a strong hold on me. I'm chained to the bar; I cannot get free.*

This made me redouble my efforts for a solution. I looked for rehab programs and cures online, but they were super expensive, so I dismissed them, rationalizing that I didn't really have a problem, and I was too good for that anyway. Yet I also felt worthless; frankly, I could not understand what was happening within me. I would later learn that was part of my insanity, feeling like an entitled perfect person, yet at the same time feeling like the worst of the worst. There was no in between.

In the back of the divorce busting book, the author recommended a marriage counseling service for alcoholic families. It gave me hope. I thought maybe I could benefit from that. I signed up. Honestly, my motivation was to show Susan how willing I was to change and how we could live happily ever after. It was an expensive six-session over-the-phone treatment program, but I was ready.

The first session, I couldn't stop crying; however, I was tipsy and drinking. I asked the counselor when my wife would join us, which was crazy to ask because I had no contact with her. The counselor said, "I don't know; maybe she won't ever join us."

I almost lost it and said, "Maybe I'll just quit this crap!" Each session I seemed to open up and discover a little more and more

STOP!

about how insane I was. Alcohol had warped my mind. After the fifth session, I accepted Susan wasn't going to join us. I realized that it was really over. And as painful as that was, I knew I would definitely die if I didn't stop drinking.

I had instinctively made a list of AA groups in my area. I thought, *just in case. I'll go there before I kill myself.*

At the end of the last phone session, my marriage counselor said, "Okay, we are done." My heart sunk. "I have a question for you," she said. "What are you going to do about your drinking? Are you going to stop, or are you just going to drink less?"

That was a very tough question for me. It was a serious question. I didn't want to commit to quitting out of fear that I wouldn't keep to my word and that I would be admitting I was powerless over alcohol. But I heard myself slowly and almost painfully saying, "I'm going to stop."

She said, "Okay, hang up the phone and get to an AA meeting that will work with the solution, not the problem." That struck me. The counseling sessions seemed to focus on good things; however, there were few. The solution was to find meetings that focused on the good things instead of only the bad things. Those words would help catapult me to just that. It was something new to me.

Lesson Learned: Focus on good things. This will help you improve and find ways to do more of those things!

Hi. My Name Is Neal, and I'm An Alcoholic

"Release the hurt, release the fear. Refuse to entertain your old pain. The energy it takes to hang on to the past is holding you back from your new life."

—Mary Manin Morrissey

As I hung up the phone, I finished my beer and thought, *this could be my last drink*. It had been approximately one month since Susan had left. I was still engulfed in darkness and didn't realize how much darker things would get. I pulled out the list and saw that I had previously circled the meeting I would attend. If I hurried, I would get there just in time for the noon meeting.

As I parked, I trembled with fear, shame, and the need to have a drink. I called a friend who had taken me to an AA meeting once before. He himself had over ten years of sobriety. He answered as if he had been waiting for my call after all this time. I immediately started crying, saying, "I'm in front of the AA group and ready to go to a meeting."

He said, "Neal, I love you! Remember, God has given you many opportunities to improve; now He's giving you another. Go to your meeting and call me once you get out."

COMFORTABLY INSANE

As I slowly opened the door, I took a deep breath. My body was bloated and at the heaviest weight I had ever been. My pants felt tight and crooked. Emotionally, the darkness had engulfed my entire being. I truly hadn't had a worse feeling than in that moment, at least I thought.

The room seemed huge, and I felt as if I had just walked into a medical facility full of happy people, laughing and smiling, and some who were just quiet. I was completely out of my element. I felt so sorry for myself for what my life had come down to.

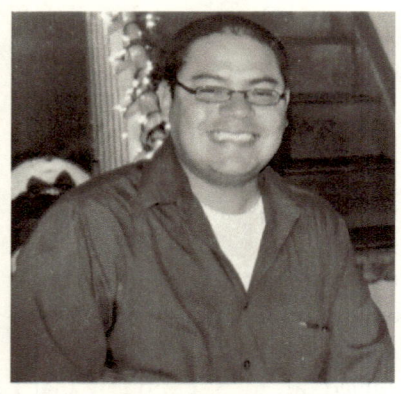

A few years before entering AA

Inside, I knew that I was there for someone else. I was there to try to impress my wife, for her to forgive me and take me back. My insanity told me that all I needed to do was remove the alcohol and life would be back to normal and happy.

I heard people talking and sharing their stories. It was a weird concept for me to understand. I mean, I related to what I was hearing, but I couldn't understand why some of the people were happy. A microphone was going around and unexpectedly made it to me.

I said, "Hi, my name is Neal, and I'm an alcoholic," merely because that was how everyone started their sharing. I dove into what was happening in my life. I recall that, at one point, I put my head down and started repeating, "I'm all alone, I'm all alone."

At this point, the facilitator said, "Neal!" I looked up, almost startled. "You're not alone anymore." When he finished saying

HI, MY NAME IS NEAL, AND I'M AN ALCOHOLIC

that, I noticed that behind him up on the wall was a quilt that said, "You're not alone." In that moment and for the first time since my wife had left the house and really for the first time in my life, I felt a momentary sense of relief. Although I was hurting badly, I wasn't alone anymore!

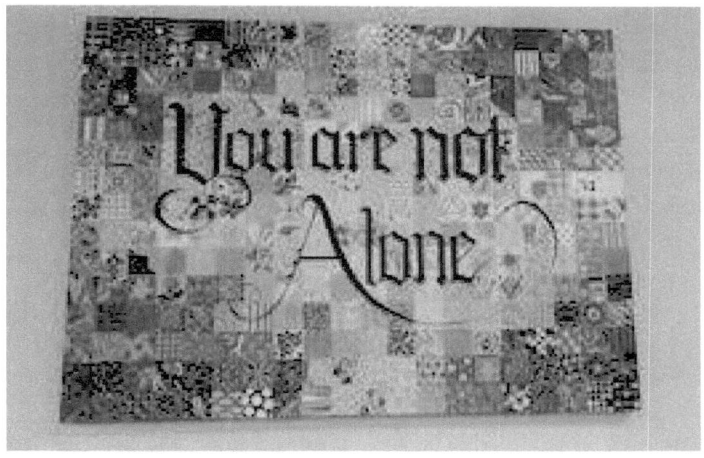

Quilt that hangs on the wall of Coral Gables Coral Room AA.

After the meeting, I was rushed with support. One guy said to me while walking out, "Neal, remember, your sobriety date is September 28, 2009." This hit me like a ton of bricks. That night, I didn't drink, although my body was begging for it and demanded the usual dosage. I couldn't sleep, and I had the sweats nonstop. While I have endured physical pain before, not being able to sleep while being alone and craving a drink has been the most trying time for me. It was hard to just sit there knowing that a drink would help me and relieve me from all those symptoms, and yet not cave to it; know that no one was around to confront or stop me from drinking. Holding myself accountable in those moments of hell helped me to grow in ways I didn't know I was looking for.

COMFORTABLY INSANE

This process repeated itself for three months. All this time, I was working really hard to keep myself sober. I was doing three meetings a day, maybe even four. On weekends, I just stayed in the AA room all day, taking notes and sharing as much as I could in meetings. I bought the AA *Big Book* and read it nonstop. The shakes were leaving me, but mental clarity wasn't coming so easily. My body responded to my constant running and pushups; however, my mind was as obsessed as ever, focusing on thoughts of the past and how I would save my marriage if I could stay sober. This insanity went from early morning to late at night. It was exhausting. In the *Big Book*, I found a chapter for the wives. I thought, *perfect! Once Susan reads it, she'll understand.* Mind you, I had read it but hadn't paid much attention to it.

Also, as I was going through this period, I was flat broke. I didn't have a penny to my name. Facing the constant threat of foreclosure and eviction from my house, I was under intense pressure.

Meanwhile, in AA, I had made a list of people to call in case I decided I wanted to drink. The instructions were that before I took a drink, I needed to call one of those people. I was on board.

One day I received a notice of the final hearing for the divorce. I had tried everything in order to reestablish the relationship. I pleaded. I begged. I called her friends, her brother, and her coworkers. I sent her flowers; I dropped letters to her house. The only person who answered in the sweetest way was her mom. She said, "Neal, get cured." She nailed it. I knew it was over. I needed to work AA.

I had even received a stern letter from her lawyer threatening legal action if I continued to reach out to her. I promptly complied. This was a painful process that taught me to stay within boundaries, as I didn't know any.

HI, MY NAME IS NEAL, AND I'M AN ALCOHOLIC

In my craziness, I viewed this notice as the perfect opportunity to state my case. I went to court that day with my best face and best intentions. I might have worn a suit. I had lost weight and my mind felt clear. After all, it had been almost three months of no alcohol. I would, however, realize I was just as insane as ever.

That day I received a good chunk of cash from work, which I thought was a sign that everything was going to turn out just fine. I energetically arrived early at the courthouse when Susan arrived. I happily asked her to sit by me as if nothing was wrong. She very calmly said, "Sure," and then sat somewhere else. She wasn't mean but just ignored me. But first, she looked deeply into my eyes. I think she was trying to see if I was hungover or maybe even drunk. Magically, she said she forgave me. I desperately needed that. When I think about it, I can't blame her at all for trying to get away from me. After all, I was trying to get away from me as well.

Once we were in front of the judge, I was ready to make my statement; however, it was done before I could say anything. Actually, it's quite annoying to me to think that I was expecting an opportunity to state my case. There was no case. It was open and shut. I was a drunk, and she wanted out!

When it was over, I walked out of there as if there was still hope. More insanity! I would describe that as passive irrationality. Not sure if that's a word or a condition.

Susan and I went down the elevator together. At first, I thought we were walking together, but really we weren't. I slowed down and she sped up. I saw her walk away. I think she might have looked back once. I leaned against a wall in the Miami courthouse, devastated. The plan hadn't worked. I did everything and more. I put 1,000 percent into this, and it didn't work!

Lesson Learned: Once the wheels of recovery are started, they never stop until you get the message. We may face death, the insane asylum, or prison if we don't take the road to recovery.

Who Are You Here For?

"I realized that anything short of being here for me wasn't going to work. I was now doing this for Neal."

—Neal Linares

I walked out of the courthouse that day completely destroyed. Then the insidious thoughts started. I live in Miami. There are so many bars open right now. Miraculously, I have plenty of money to do whatever I want in terms of drinking. That thought engulfed my entire being. Almost with glee, I declared I could get a drink; after all, I had the perfect excuse. I just got a divorce. It was decided: I would drink! I just had to find a bar. It would most likely be an all-day thing and perhaps even an all-week thing, but for now, all I had to worry about was getting to the bar and putting myself into a state of oblivion. It was quite relieving to know that I didn't have to fake sobriety anymore. She was gone. I had lost.

On this bright, sunny mid-morning, I was in front of the metro rail station. I sat down on a bench around a fountain to gather myself for a moment. I soon noticed I was surrounded by homeless people. I was struck by how hopeless they looked. I wondered what happened in their lives that caused them to end up here. A lost job? A tragic event, like divorce? An addiction or a mental illness? That thought made me think of my future and where I would end up if I drank again. But surely, it couldn't do me any harm if I did it just one more time. Then I remembered the phone numbers I had so diligently saved in AA. I pulled out my list and thought, *okay, call and then go drink just as instructed*. I picked a number from the list and called. A deep voice answered. I said, "Hey, this is Neal from the group. I just got divorced. I'm in downtown Miami. I've decided I'm going to drink and am making the phone call I was told to make before I drink."

He said, "Oh, yes." He seemed to know me. "Okay, good. Do you have a minute?"

I said, "Of course." In my mind, there was absolutely nothing he could say to soothe me or calm me or change my mind. It just wasn't possible.

He proceeded to tell me his story, which I won't share here because it's his. As he continued to share and share, I found myself having to stand and then take a seat several times. I was full of rage, fear, and anxiety. One of the homeless guys, with a look of desperation, interrupted my phone call to ask me for money. I reacted with comradery. I promptly searched in my pockets and gave him some money while internally saying, *I am one of you, my friend*.

I continued listening to my friend. His story was so powerful. It was similar to mine; I felt connected. I listened, and then something that I can only describe as a miracle happened. I didn't want to go and drink. Maybe it was even that feeling of being watched over and protected that I had felt before. Something greater than me stopped me that day from taking a drink—that and the man from AA who took the time to talk to me when I called. This was one of the first of many miracles to come. About forty minutes later, he stopped. I had cried the whole time he was sharing.

WHO ARE YOU HERE FOR?

He said, "Are you there?"

With a trembling voice, I said, "Yes."

"Have you changed your mind? Can you make it to a meeting?"

"Yes."

I was so amazed at the mental shift. I had never changed my mind once I had decided to drink. It just wasn't possible for me to do that.

On my way to the meeting, the thought came to me, *who are you going to this meeting for?* I realized I had been going to meetings for my second ex-wife, my parents, my business, my first ex-wife, and my son. I realized that all this time, I had attended for everyone else but me. I somberly walked into the room and sat quietly. I drifted in and out of crying and feeling completely sorry for myself. I was thinking about earlier in the courthouse when my ex-wife had said she forgave me. As I was thinking of this, someone handed me the microphone. "My name is Neal. I'm an alcoholic, and I just came from the courthouse where I just got a divorce."

Everyone cheered and exclaimed, "D day."

I was startled. I continued sharing. "Despite everything, I feel good because she said she forgave me."

Before the meeting ended, I saw this guy stand up and make his way up to me. He always described himself as an alcoholic with a slight cocaine problem. He leaned in and whispered in my ear, "Now you just have to learn to forgive yourself." That one hit me like a ton of bricks. What was he talking about? What does that even mean?

COMFORTABLY INSANE

That night, I didn't drink. I was definitely at a crossroads. I knew, deep down in my heart, that this was the true beginning of my journey.

I kept asking myself, *who are you here for? What are you trying to do? Why do you want to be sober?* I had read the AA book from cover to cover, and I had no answers.

> **Lesson Learned:** Sobriety requires that you undertake the journey for yourself. Only then can you turn around and help others.

I'm Sick

"The two most important days of your life are when you are born and when you know why."

—Mark Twain

As each day passed, my thoughts and emotions were becoming a little clearer and more in check. I was beginning to understand how wrong my thought patterns were and how insane I had become; however, healing this would take longer than I could ever imagine.

One day I decided to sit down and reread every word of the chapter to the wives in the AA book. I realized that the first time I tried to read this chapter that in my excitement to get it to Susan, I barely read it. I simply made copies and passed them to her almost with an attitude of arrogance, as if saying, "There. Read; that will explain everything. You just need to understand the deal."

This time I wanted to read it slowly, to digest it word for word in hopes of figuring out why my marriage had not worked. I got to a point where it described how alcoholics have caused tremendous pain to their family, wives, children, employers, and many others. It went on to say, "Although they have all suffered, they have not suffered more than the alcoholics themselves." This sentence hit me like a ton of bricks.

COMFORTABLY INSANE

I stopped, and for the first time, I said to myself, "I'm sick!" My dad had recently been diagnosed with cancer, and I, for some reason, correlated the two. Just like he needs treatment, I need treatment, and I knew my illness was just as deadly as his. I was suffering, and that was okay because if I treat this as a disease, I can get well!

Lesson Learned: Alcoholism or addiction is a disease. If I treat it that way, then and only then can I get better.

The Twenty-Year First Step

*"We admitted we were powerless over alcohol—
that our lives had become unmanageable."*

—Step One, *AA*

I was now thirty-eight years old, and for the first time since I had sat in that rehab center as a teenager listening to the kids declare they were powerless over alcohol, I too found myself saying, "I'm powerless over alcohol." It had taken more than twenty years of emotional and physical destruction to get there.

I felt that thing/power that had protected me all my life was also trying to teach me. And for the first time in my life, I started to connect some of the dots of my behaviors. I felt empowered.

I wasn't concerned anymore about why it had taken so long to understand. I was just humbled. It seemed that I had finally found the door to the solution. Maybe, just maybe, this could be the beginning of a happy, peaceful life. I could see it. More importantly, I could feel it!

Finally, a real feeling!

My heart was full, and for the first time, I thought, *I'm so grateful to be an alcoholic. I have hope!*

Lesson Learned: Experience is the true teacher of understanding why things happen.

The Business and My Dad

"Transformation is often more about unlearning than learning."

—Richard Rohr

Ever since the day I made the decision to work for the family business as a teenager after high school, I had worked extremely hard. This business felt like the heart of the family, with my dad as the pillar. When we first started, we had so much hope and desire. Through the years, we had squashed every fear with pure grit, determination, and action. It seemed, for such a long time, that nothing could stop us. My brother and mother also worked with us. And, at one point or another, all of my sisters had had their time in the business. After more than twenty years, it had taken a toll on me. The fact that my dad was now sick with cancer made it even harder.

The family business was hurting and had been hurting for quite a while. The economy had taken a turn for the worse in 2008, and in 2009, we were hanging on for dear life; however, we had the gift of not quitting no matter how bad things were. This proved to be a gift and a curse at the same time.

COMFORTABLY INSANE

We had a machine that we had put all our resources into, but it never functioned properly. We later suspected it had been dropped or something. After many repairs, it broke down for the final time. We had no more resources, and for the first time, accepted that we had to quit.

As this was happening, our dad was fighting cancer in another state. He was spared from handling any of the final closing business arrangements. It was quite a difficult moment, and yet at the same time, it was liberating because I had felt that pressure for many years.

A big part of my relationship with my dad came from being in business with him. Since his cancer prevented him from being actively involved in the business, I made a few visits to connect with him. We both regretted missing opportunities to connect when I was younger. As a kid, I participated in the Cub Scouts pinewood derby program. I made a car by myself that sucked. I couldn't figure out how to carve the wood block. Though I tried my best, the car barely rolled. I had wished my dad could have helped with that car, but that was a time when he wasn't around much because of work. During one of our many phone conversations, he shared with me that he recently had an opportunity to serve in church working with the Cub Scouts. They were participating in the pinewood derby, and my dad decided to make his own car. His turned out to be the fastest car in the unofficial races. His experience brought me back to the time when I tried making my own car so very long ago. I would have loved his help. Listening to him share this made me so jealous and so happy at the same time.

THE BUSINESS AND MY DAD

Lesson Learned: When fighting alcohol or addiction, material things and past regrets cannot matter. The only thing that matters is staying sober.

Working My Recovery

"Our human resources, as marshalled by the will, were not sufficient; they failed utterly . . . Every day is a day when we must carry the vision of God's will into all our activities."

—*Alcoholics Anonymous*, pp. 45, 85

I was so busy working and going to AA meetings. Because I went to so many, I often needed my parents to babysit my son while I went. I had become addicted to those meetings, but anything was better than drinking.

I remember, though, needing something more than just meetings. So the same AA philosophy suggested I find a good church to go to, and being LDS, I agreed, but I wasn't ready to take action just yet.

However hopeful I was at this time, I suffered greatly from feelings of depression—as strong as ever. One day, these feelings were at an all-time high. The previous night, I had watched a show about a guy who was trying to kill himself. His idea was to run himself to death. I thought that since I ran and I also loved to run in the high Miami heat, I would try it too! It was settled. The committee, what I dubbed my thoughts that I listened to, decided we would go out running, and maybe, if we got lucky, I wouldn't come back.

COMFORTABLY INSANE

It was blazing hot, and the sun was as intense as ever; however, as I went out for my run, the sky became cloudy. The heat was gone. I ran and ran and finally realized I wasn't going to die. I returned and sat in my living room defeated. As I sat there, a ray of sunshine hit my face through the window. I felt this overwhelming peace and comfort fill my body. It was as if God himself had winked at me. I tried to soak it in as much as possible. After a moment, I decided to get the mail to feel more of the sun. There I found a letter from some bishop I had never met before. In a nutshell, the letter said, "If you're hurting and are looking for peace, come. We can help; we welcome you." I was angry. I felt like a cornered or wounded animal that someone is trying to help, but the animal instead bites back. Assuming it was my mom's doing, I called her and asked her to please not ask anyone from church to contact me.

She calmly said, "I haven't called anyone, so maybe it's a sign that you should go to church." When she said that, I again got that feeling of peace and serenity. Next Sunday, I was at church.

I sat in the back pew and didn't want to talk to anyone. I sat there and cried. It was hard to be there. Everything seemed so reverent and good. I felt so irreverent and ugly. But it was harder not to be there. I hadn't taken a drink for over three months and my dark feelings seemed to have intensified rather than gotten better.

Going back to church gave me so many new tools to combat my depression, the desire to drink, and the feelings of being lost in life. Church was and still is a huge part of my life.

During this time, the committee and I decided I would go back to school to finish a bachelor's degree.

At thirty-eight years old and after several previous years of community college, I was accepted to Florida International University. I remember this day vividly. You see, I had been rejected before. It seemed as if my mindset was one of never being able to accomplish. I had friends and family who had graduated, but even though I considered myself capable, I thought I wasn't fit for school. That was very ironic and definitely a false belief. I cried as I read the letter of acceptance. I now had a new goal and purpose.

Lesson Learned: Being sober did not mean that my darkness would be lifted. In fact, it may intensify as we transition to the light.

The Blitz

"AA taught me not to be overwhelmed, but rather to accept and understand my life as it unfolded."

—*AA Daily Reflections*, p. 174

Post-divorce blues, foreclosure, family court, bankruptcy, school, work, and all the business issues that needed attention were starting to drown me.

This was definitely not the best time to add school to the mix. Just one of those problems alone is enough to have your plate full. When I think back, I truly don't know how I got through such a barrage of serious issues. Even though all this was happening, staying sober was my number one priority. I proactively would ask myself what lesson I should learn in each situation I encountered, and as such, I only saw the good in everything. At the time, I was flat out broke and had no money for lawyers. But I needed a lawyer for a number of things.

Around this time, I became very close with a friend and new mentor from church. He had some knowledge about the justice system because he had had experiences with his own home.

COMFORTABLY INSANE

He helped me with my legal representation for my house. During one of the shares at an AA meeting, I said, "I accept that I will have to leave my house, and I'm okay."

When I got out of the meeting, I had five missed calls. It was my friend from church. He said, "Neal, I think I can help you with your house." He then asked if he could look at the mortgage papers. I agreed, more out of respect because I didn't believe there was anything he could do. I took the papers to his house where he reviewed them. He quickly found discrepancies, and I set out to clear them up in the courts.

The very first time I went to court, I was scared out of my mind. My first AA sponsor happened to be a lawyer and had agreed to help me. Also, another dear AA friend was a court reporter and had agreed to transcribe the hearing. Come to think of it, this girl had given me my white chip in the AA meeting. To me, she was an angel. I remember getting there and shaking with fear. I'm not sure if it was visible to others, but inside I was barely making it. The result of this hearing would determine if I had to leave my house or if I could stay.

I sat in the courtroom waiting for my turn. Finally the case came up. I respectfully walked up with my sponsor, who began stating the case with me filling in the blanks as needed. The other party didn't have the answers to our questions. We had caught them off guard. Even my sponsor was surprised. In an amazing turn of events, the judge overturned the final summary judgment and asked the prosecution to please answer the questions and the pending papers. I was elated, although I really didn't understand what had happened. I turned to my sponsor, who saw the confusion on my face and said, "You don't realize what just happened, do you? Well let me put it this way. Imagine that you're in the last game in the World Series. Bases are loaded at the bottom of the ninth inning with two outs and full count, and the only way you win is with a home run. And you just hit it! You just hit a home run! You don't have to give up your house." It was so exciting. That cemented my trust in my new friend and mentors from church and the AA groups.

That night, sitting in my house, I tried to understand this change of good fortune and what I had done to deserve good supportive friends. I had a mind shift that day. It was okay to ask for and receive help. For the first time in my life, I felt good people around me. All they wanted was to help. Nothing else.

After many court hearings, I eventually did lose the battle for my house. But it was five years before I had to leave, and having the security of somewhere to live for those five years was priceless. I remember one time in preparation for foreclosure, I had gotten rid of all the furniture I had, including my bed. A friend had suggested that I learn to be grateful. I called her the next morning and said, "I'm grateful because I didn't have to make the bed this morning."

We both laughed.

At this same time, I had a contentious family case from my first marriage that took so much energy. Since I had contributed to these problems, it was important I took responsibility for my actions and learned to make things right. But I was used to giving in and being walked over because I felt so guilty about my past actions. Yes, I needed to take ownership for my mistakes, but I also needed to remember I was not responsible for the actions of others. But by guilt alone, I was doing that. I had been accustomed to making decisions on my guilty feelings, and therefore, I absorbed all the faults to be my own. While most of them were my fault, I started to digest this idea that I was not responsible for the actions of others. This gave me a little bit of breathing room, as well as the desire to push back just a bit. Because of a lack of money, I was also my own lawyer in this case.

COMFORTABLY INSANE

For some reason, this chapter is harder than others—I think maybe because there were so many things getting ironed out in my life and in my mind. The same AA friend whom I had called right before going into my first meeting said to me, "It's beautiful to see someone bouncing at the bottom of the barrel." Of course, he was referring to me. I thought, *holy crap! I'm at the bottom of the barrel!*

Angrily, I asked, "And how is that?"

With a smile, he said, "Well, as you're slowly stripped of all your old ideas and misconceptions of yourself, you'll adopt new ones that will lift you and make you a better person as you climb out of the bottom of the barrel."

I thought it was the dumbest thing I had ever heard! But at the same time, I had no other choice than to accept it to be true. If not, nothing made sense. So, after a year of sobriety, I found myself at the bottom of the barrel. Or so I thought.

It never crossed my mind that there were barrels within barrels and more bottoms to come.

Lesson Learned: I am much stronger than I think. For each situation where I feel defenseless and helpless, if I am humble, that can turn into strength.

Step Five and the Bus

"Admitted to God, to ourselves, and to another human being the exact nature of our wrongs."

—AA Step Five

As I was feeling the full power of the blitz, I received a letter notifying me that my license would be suspended until I paid a fine for back child support. I simply didn't have the money. I had so many things going on: the foreclosure case, the family court case, and my personal bankruptcy case. Additionally, I was studying full time and working.

I spoke to my second AA sponsor about this problem. You see, I had changed sponsors because my first one was giving me too much trouble with my fourth step. Bottom line: I didn't want to do the work.

My sponsor and I decided that the safest route to take would be for me to continue driving, but to do so safely and go through the back roads to avoid police. After all, I had way too much to take care of. Simultaneously, I had friends from the groups who were 100 percent opposed to that idea. I thought about it and made my decision. I was going to continue driving. One day, as I was carefully driving from a client's office, I was at a stoplight, and

COMFORTABLY INSANE

BAM! I got rear-ended. I panicked and froze for a few seconds. But the driver, a young kid, reversed and took off. As I heard their tires screech, I snapped out of it and called my sponsor. He told me to get the hell out of there. So I did.

If there had been any police officers at the scene, from what I was told, it would have been twenty-one days in jail for driving without a license. I had just started a brand-new semester, and I had court hearings to attend to. It would have caused more chaos in my life than what I was already experiencing. But after that incident, I reversed the decision of driving without a license. Ha! I was not going to risk it. I would not be driving anymore. This decision, however, put me in a very difficult situation. In the area I lived in at the time, public transportation wasn't the best. I was pretty bitter that I had to deal with all the issues on my plate, and now, I had no car. The first day of this new routine, I got my books and sales presentation ready in time to leave at four-thirty in the morning to make the 6:15 a.m. bus that would take me to school. From school, I would catch another bus that would take me either to downtown Miami or Coral Gables, a city next to Miami. I had to be very selective with my clients now, and sometimes had to choose them solely by bus routes. This went on for five months. Sometimes, it was school, court, and clients. Other times, it was school, court, and AA meetings. It was always an adventure, especially when I mistakenly got on the wrong bus and ended up somewhere different.

When my car was taken away from me, I was bitter. I realized how spoiled I was when I could drive to my AA meetings in the comfort of my car, arrive, get my treats, have an amazing meeting, jump back in the car again, and drive back to my house.

I woke up every morning not knowing how the day was going to roll out. One time, I remember getting ready in a suit and tie because I had an important client conference. I took my books for

STEP FIVE AND THE BUS

school and jumped on the bus. I arrived at the meeting just in time. When I left and walked to the bus stop, it started pouring rain. I couldn't believe it. Sadly, this wouldn't be the last time I got soaked.

However, it seemed as if a miracle were brewing. Each day, a sense of peace was descending upon me. I could feel it. As time wore on, I would wake up at four-thirty in the morning and get ready to hurriedly walk to the bus. I no longer felt so bitter. This change came after three months of doing this bus routine. It was fascinating to me how my mind and emotions had shifted. The actual trial of not having a car had made things so difficult but had also caused me to look for solutions and find the good. I was excited to find them each day.

I was also practicing asking for help. I asked friends for rides. Sometimes, I got them; sometimes, I didn't. A few times, I got stood up. But the cool thing was that I could now ask without expecting anything in return. Well, to a certain point. I was, and still am, very human, and rejection hurts a bit. But I didn't feel sorry for myself or get angry anymore. This was something new to me.

This reminded me of a story about a guy who was so cheerful all the time. His neighbor, whenever he saw him, would say, "Mr. So and So, spring's in the air," and this guy had such a great attitude that he would literally spring in the air! I couldn't believe it, but I was starting to feel that way. I was working hard to get things done. But during those early morning walks to catch the bus, I felt like springing in the air. It was truly miraculous to experience. My heart and mind were changing.

One time, I had family court and a calculus exam on the same day. I had studied for both the court case and the calculus exam for countless hours. I still didn't have money for lawyers, so I represented myself and learned how to do things from the internet. That day, I made it to court, presented my case, and was surprised by how well I did. Internally, I realized I had very negative feelings about court ever since my teenage years. They plagued me without my awareness; however, my mindset at the time was to spring in the air no matter what.

I ran to the bus after court, feeling super stressed about the exam. I got to class just in time. I did my very best but ended up failing that exam. Later, I failed the entire class. The professor explained that I would have been better off missing that first exam. He said he could have passed me because of my average. I couldn't believe it. But, amazingly, I wasn't angry or bitter! Truly amazing! Amongst all the difficulty, I was learning to let go and accept things as they were. It would be okay. Everything would be okay and work out no matter what, as long as I did not cling to any outcomes and did my best

Even with all this positivity, I did have some anxiety still, especially when home alone. The day before I got rear-ended, I had prayed and fasted for help with my anxiety over being alone, asking to be able to overcome this anxiety and sleep well. In the past, this had always proven to be impossible. Taking naps was also out of the question. I always had to be moving, like I was running away from something. I would always jump at any opportunity that required leaving the house. Without a car, that became difficult. More and more, I found myself having to stay inside the house.

This was so difficult in the beginning, as I was bitter and hurt, but with time, I overcame this as well. One time I invited the missionaries from church over for dinner, not because I wanted to but rather because I was dying inside. I thought maybe if I did something that I perceived to be good, I'd feel better. I didn't have any food or groceries. So I jumped on the bike, rode to the store, and bought the things I needed and made them food. It was a lot of effort. But I needed to do it more for me. I did feel better. It was a wonderful evening.

STEP FIVE AND THE BUS

Financially, I was a mess. I mustered up the courage and asked my bishop for help. He made it so painless and agreed to drop off some food on Tuesday. As Tuesday arrived, I waited anxiously since I had nothing to eat. I waited and waited. He never showed. Later that evening, he called me apologetically and said he had forgotten and that he would stop by on Thursday. I was embarrassed and grateful. Oh, and very hungry! I had to dig deep and eventually found some cans of food around the house. I was learning not to take things personally, to always accept that things would be okay, and overall, to be grateful for everything that came my way. Good or bad.

Bitterness had turned into joy as I slowly let go of my old life, losing people, places, and things. When I look back, I wouldn't change one single thing. Well, maybe one thing. I would definitely have changed my ability to learn the concept of "let go" sooner and quicker.

The miracle was that after this blitz, I found what seemed to be the beginning of peace and serenity. This was something I had never felt before. I could now see how living a sober life was possible. It felt like I was understanding who I was and how being responsible meant not being responsible for the world but for myself. As a consequence, everything else would take care of itself.

Exercising was crucial in my sobriety. Running had become a passion. Yup, I had picked this up from military school. And thankfully, I no longer had to run in the dark morning full of potholes or with an angry sergeant beating me with a bamboo stick.

I could feel my whole body when I ran. The committee was in full swing when I ran. I would let my thoughts run completely loose with a million ideas and plans. The committee was always so loud, but as I ran and ran, it would always transform, and still does to this day, into a soothing conversation. It was powerful!

COMFORTABLY INSANE

Often, when I reached levels of exhaustion on my run, I would start to cry. I knew deep down that this was healing me. It was pushing me to access both physical and spiritual levels that I had never reached before. It developed my patience. It allowed me to trust others, but most importantly, it opened the door to my inner self, to understand that I could do and learn hard things and come out on top.

I was working on step five with my sponsor at this time. Step five is a powerful and vulnerable step. It asks one to "admit to God, to ourselves, and to another human being the exact nature of our wrongs."

My sponsor and I had gone to a peaceful park. In what seemed like three to four hours, I told him everything, except the incident in El Salvador with the dudes. As we were leaving, I was overcome with fear that if I didn't tell him everything, I would drink again. I stopped and said, "Hey, I still need to tell you something." We sat again, and I let it out. He listened. When I was finished, he said, "Neal, I love you! That incident doesn't define you." Later, I realized my personal accountability for that incident. Of course it wasn't all my fault, but I had to take some responsibility since no one had forced me to get on the bus to go there. I went on my own. True, I had been tricked into the situation and, for that, I wasn't responsible. I could only take responsibility for my actions, not for the actions of others.

I went home with the weight of the world removed and took a long nap, feeling completely at peace.

STEP FIVE AND THE BUS

Lesson Learned: My higher power reaches inside my soul to answer my prayers. He knows every crevasse of my weaknesses, and he tailor-makes lessons that only I could personally understand for my improvement.

Trudging the Road of Sobriety

"Abandon yourself to God as you understand God. Admit your faults to Him and to your fellows. Clear away the wreckage of your past. Give freely of what you find and join us. We shall be with you in the Fellowship of the Spirit, and you will surely meet some of us as you trudge the Road of Happy Destiny. May God bless you and keep you—until then."

—*AA Book*, p. 164

Sometimes, I've thought that because I've experienced so many hardships and somehow have overcome, my life now will be better and easier.

I remember many times thinking, *I'm not drinking. Why are things not better? Why does everything have to be so hard for me?* This thought process, of course, implied that everyone else had it easy.

Many times, I witnessed people start AA, and in a matter of months, their wives had taken them back, they were financially stable, their messy lives seemed to clean up quickly, and everything was okay. For me, it had been three years of sobriety, yet things were still heavy and messy. Although I had had tremendous breakthroughs—like taking peaceful naps at home and taking responsibility for my own actions—overall, I felt I just couldn't get ahead. Depression and insanity had been my lifelong companion. I realized that these feelings were my comfort zone more than ever. I found the idea of being crazy comforting. It protected me. It gave me an excuse. Alcohol provided that excuse for me. Now that it was removed, I had no excuses for failing or for being depressed. It was very uncomfortable. I noticed when things were going well, while it excited me, I also felt uncomfortable. It was so foreign to me that, at times, I would subconsciously find conflict. I continued connecting the dots and noticed patterns. Conflict made me feel comfortable. It was what I knew. It was my safety.

In retrospect, this was my pattern: work hard at finding something that made me happy, enjoy it for a little bit until I felt it was secured, then destroy it. This insight has proven valuable as I've caught myself in the middle or end of the pattern many times and, sometimes, have even been able to change course.

This thought process fell right in line with my experience with the *Big Book* of AA, page 114. This is the chapter about the wives and families of alcoholics, which I mentioned before. Here it is word for word. I feel it's worth citing in full once again: "The wives and children suffer horribly, but not more than the men themselves."

This very sentence changed my life once before, and now when I read it again, it cemented something in my soul. As an alcoholic, I was sick. Just like someone who's sick needs treatment, so did I. This concept was truly liberating for me. It allowed me to work as hard as I humanly could on my well-being. It helped me live, knowing that I might see beautiful cases of life in a gloomy or skewed perspective. I learned that I was always thinking, *when is this happy moment going to go bad?* It was so deep inside that only the idea of being sick helped to bring it to the forefront and let it out!

TRUDGING THE ROAD OF SOBRIETY

Lesson Learned: Sobriety doesn't mean instant happiness, perfection, or bliss. It rather means facing things without the filter of alcohol. You become unmasked.

I'm Cured?

"He who is born a fool is never cured."

—Proverb

I devised a new physical workout plan that helped me succeed with my schoolwork. Whenever I could, I'd go for long runs to settle my nerves just before exams. I needed the mental patience it gave me, especially when taking algebra and calculus. They were my foes. It turned out that I really liked both these subjects, but I sucked at them and had deep issues. I harbored either resentment or fear—honestly not sure which—with math that stemmed from when I was a kid. Whatever it was, it was cemented even deeper down while I was in military school.

As a result of this, I took algebra four times in college before I passed and ended up taking calculus two times. The first time I failed calculus, I was broken and sad. I called my dad and told him I failed and didn't know if I had it in me to try again. He listened quietly.

At this time, my relationship with my dad had been repaired.

After a while, he asked, "What are you going to do?"

I paused. "I'm going to enroll and try again."

COMFORTABLY INSANE

He said, "That's my boy!"

It was exactly what I needed to hear. I immediately enrolled and attacked that class like there was no tomorrow. This second time I was more determined than ever. With that effort of sheer determination and the kindness of my professor, I had a chance. I set a meeting with the new professor. I told her my experience with the last class and that I had failed.

She advised me to work really hard, and when I no longer could figure it out on my own, then and only then should I get a tutor.

I really appreciated this advice because the first time around, I had paid for a tutor and still failed, so this helped me realize I was making good decisions, which meant maybe I was cured.

Halfway through the semester, I was holding my own. I was getting low grades on the exams and quizzes, but I was giving it my all and making sure my professor knew. For every answer I couldn't figure out on a test or quiz, I would write a little note, explaining the process so she knew I understood. I felt I was in a war to pass and everything counted.

One weekend while sitting with one of my best friends from recovery at a coffee shop, my cell phone rang. And there it was. The call I was hoping never to receive. It was my older sister.

"Dad has four weeks or less to live," she said somberly.

I couldn't breathe; it was as though an elephant had stepped on me. I couldn't take the pressure of the class and my dad dying. It was unbearable. I didn't cry but quickly put on one of my masks from within and told those around me that I was fine.

Later that night, it hit me. I cried and cried.

I'M CURED?

It was so unfair. I was supposed to enjoy and develop a better relationship with my dad when he got better. When I got better. When we got better. We were a team, two sick dudes getting better, waiting for that victory!

I knew there were so many things he wished he would have done differently with his children as they grew up. But now with my new discoveries of alcoholics, I felt I knew him and understood him much better. Perhaps even more than he himself understood.

Armed with my new knowledge of AA, I recognized some of my dad's character flaws as those of an alcoholic. I was learning to deal with them. At first, I felt horrible because I felt he never did. But then when analyzing his life transformation, I realized he did in his own way. That gave me comfort.

One time, when I had just started my path to sobriety, I called and screamed at him over the phone.

"Where were you? All those times when I needed you! Where were you when horrible things were happening to me?"

He quietly listened and let me scream on and on, releasing all my anger and frustrations from when I was a kid, from military school to the current moment and everything in between. He just listened.

When I had nothing else to say, he very softly said, "I'm here now."

In that moment, all my anger and frustration toward him vanished. Those words filled my heart with love and peace. I never had to question him again because I understood what he meant. He could do absolutely nothing about the past. But now he was there to listen and help me as I needed.

I thought maybe I would buy a scout derby car kit and we could make one together before he passed away.

I was trying to coordinate a trip, but I was flat broke. There was no way I could fly. I was about to give up when my sweet cousin offered to help by providing the tickets for both my brother and me. We were so grateful.

This meant I would have to withdraw from calculus. The way I was feeling, I was seriously considering withdrawing from all of school and just calling it quits to the whole bachelor's degree. I went to the offices and put in my request to drop the class. The higher power or angel that has always helped me was there again. I could feel it. I walked up to the desk and spoke with a young girl whose name I will never know and who I will likely never see again.

When I told her I was there to withdraw from my calculus class, she took my info and said, "Hey, you're almost done with your degree. But you failed this class once before. If you fail it again, you're going to be in trouble."

I explained, "My dad is dying, and I have to fly out to see him."

She stopped looking at the screen, looked straight in my eyes, and sternly but warmly said, "Hey, go take care of your dad. Come back and finish the class. Don't withdraw."

I was startled. I mean, she was maybe eighteen or so. But I just looked back at her and knew she was right. I found myself mumbling in consent. I walked out of there stunned. I looked at the time and saw that calculus class was starting in a few minutes. I snapped out of it and ran! For some reason, running to class felt normal. Out of the blue, I had new resolve. I decided to pass the class.

I'M CURED?

I took notes and listened intently. After the class, I told the professor what was going on. She strongly suggested I drop the class.

I told her that wasn't an option and asked what I could do.

She gave me the assignments, and that was it.

The next day, I went to my regular noon AA meeting in an emotional state. The guy at the concession asked me what was wrong.

I told him all that was going on: my class, my dad, all of it. He was quiet.

After the meeting, he said to me, "Hey, Neal, you still feeling sorry for yourself?"

I was offended for a second. Then I realized I was in a much bigger war. Much bigger than calculus or my dad dying. My biggest war was to stay sober. I was getting dangerously close to that drink. I was grateful for that dude and my AA family.

On the plane flying to Utah, I decided that if my dad died, I would get drunk on the way back. Another insane thought.

In Utah, I immediately went to the hospital to be at my dad's side. We exchanged a few words, and I told him I loved him. Over the next days, I watched my dad suffer from intense pain and then wither away. Everyone in the family was taking shifts to watch him. When it wasn't my turn, I was in the waiting area working on my calculus. I knew that my dad wanted that. It gave me strength.

I remember two significant exchanges with him during that time. In one, he came to, and I had him sign a do not resuscitate paper, which said that if his heart stopped beating he did not want to be resuscitated due to his condition.

In the second exchange, I'm not sure if it was all in my mind, but when he was knocked out, I kissed his forehead, leaned in, and said, "I love you; it's okay to let go. Rest in Jesus."

I swear I heard him say, "I love you too."

At that point, to me, my dad was gone. I had said my goodbye, and I was prepared for the rest.

This proved to be such an emotional and heavy goodbye that I had to leave the hospital. I needed to be alone. I got into the car and drove. I knew I needed to call my sponsor back in Miami. He listened. I said, "I'm trying to work my program. I'm trying to stay sober, but life is too much for me; I cannot handle—"

"You're not trying! You're fucking doing it! Take care of your dad and come home and do what you need to do," he said.

It has been advice and a bit of reality like this that have carried me through the roughest parts of sobriety. My dad passed January 27, 2012. It was hard. It was painful. As we were going through his belongings, I decided all I wanted was the pinewood derby car he had made. I got it!

I went home, and guess what. I didn't drink on the plane!

I continued my efforts in calculus. After the final, a few days later the professor called me in. She was a very kind lady from Haiti. She sympathized with me. She regretfully informed me that I had not passed the final. I took a long pause as I soaked the information in. She then very firmly said, "But you passed my class." I almost cried and wanted to hug her. I felt that extra effort of writing little notes on the exams and quizzes, of turning in every assignment, and of communicating closely with her had paid off.

I'M CURED?

I learned there was no easy, quick cure. Just reprieves. I bought a reflections book from AA. It's full of inspiring AA quotes and sayings for every day of the year. The page dated September 24, a random date, soon became my warning and my comfort . . .

"Today, I'm an alcoholic. Tomorrow will be no different. My alcoholism lives in me now and forever. I must never forget what I am. Alcohol will surely kill me if I fail to recognize and acknowledge my disease on a daily basis. I'm not playing a game in which a loss is a temporary setback. I'm dealing with my disease, for which there's no cure, only daily acceptance and vigilance."

—*AA Daily Reflections*, p. 276

Lesson Learned: "Vigilance: We have seen the truth demonstrated again and again. 'Once an alcoholic, always an alcoholic.' Commencing to drink after a period of sobriety, we are in a short time as bad as ever. If we are planning to stop drinking, there must be no reservation of any kind, nor any lurking notion that someday we will be immune to alcohol."
AA p. 33

Graduation! Happily Never After

"Happiness does not depend on what you have or who you are, it solely relies on what you think."

—Unknown

When I got home from Utah, I felt changed. I knew I had missed the opportunity of my life to connect and develop my relationship with my dad during my growing years. It was hard. While I was committed to being sober, I wasn't entirely happy. I was always under the impression that if I ever was able to stop drinking, my life would be happy! Everything would fall into place. Instead of my life falling into place, what I got was my dad passing away, a slew of legal cases, and feelings of despair that I had never felt before with such clarity. I didn't have a buffer anymore. And to clarify, I had felt despair before, but these were unknown levels. This was truly reaching lower and deeper into my soul.

I was at the bottom of the barrel again, but it just felt I was even further down than ever before. By this time, I had my driving privileges back; however, I wasn't able to afford my car, and it was soon repossessed. I again told myself I didn't care. It didn't faze me. Nothing did anymore. I had learned to accept and let go for the most part. But I still felt despair and grief. It took effort. Despite these feelings, I plowed through the last semesters of

COMFORTABLY INSANE

college. I say plowed because I knew nothing was going to stop me. During this whole time, I was constantly studying, whether it was cooped up in the house, at the university library, or on the bus. Every chance I got, I pulled a book out and studied. It's funny how alcoholics sometimes get accused of not having a strong will. An alcoholic, on a mission, is unstoppable. The unfortunate thing is that, most of the time, they're on a mission to drink. But a recovering alcoholic possesses the strongest will I have ever seen.

Graduation came. I had finally arrived at my graduation date, May 13, 2012. I had made it in spite of foreclosure, family court, a super hard time with algebra and calculus, no car, no money, bankruptcy court, divorce, closing the business, and my father passing away. And not to mention all while fighting the biggest battle of trying to stay sober. It was truly a miracle. I now knew who had been protecting me: God! No doubts, no confusion, I just knew. I was so grateful. My family rallied to support me that day. They flew in from Utah. While I was so happy to have them, I still felt lonely inside.

The actual graduation took place in the university's basketball arena. When my name was called, I heard my mom scream, "Yay, Neal!"

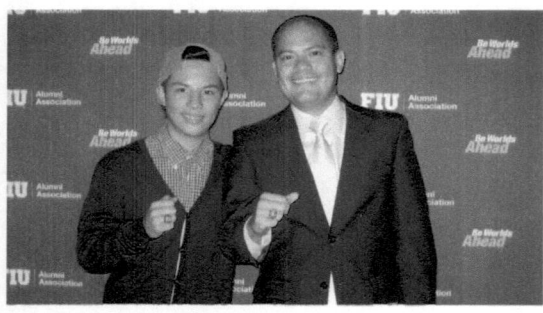

My son Zach and I at graduation.

It transported me back to when I was a little kid playing little league baseball back in North Salt Lake. When I was up to bat, my mom was always screaming the loudest, showing her support. That was my mom, always cheering me on. The

GRADUATION! HAPPILY NEVER AFTER

love of a mom is truly one of the biggest miracles. I've been able to appreciate this more in sobriety. Many times, when I hit emotional lows, I go to her for her support to pull me through. I call her my secret weapon.

After the celebration and with my family gone, I was in the house feeling alone and experiencing another round of depression.

It was always a battle of highs and lows. While I was able to keep my house for longer than I thought, I eventually got the eviction notice. It was another blow. But I was ready. I got the important things out of the house and left. I was able to rent a small room in a house, an efficiency—that's what they call it in Miami. I felt so out of place. A few days later, I got a call from the security guard from the gated community I had just been evicted from. We had become friends, and I looked at her almost as my grandma.

She said, very worried, "Neal, they threw out all your stuff. It's all flying everywhere. It's all over the lawn and street. If you hurry, you can save it."

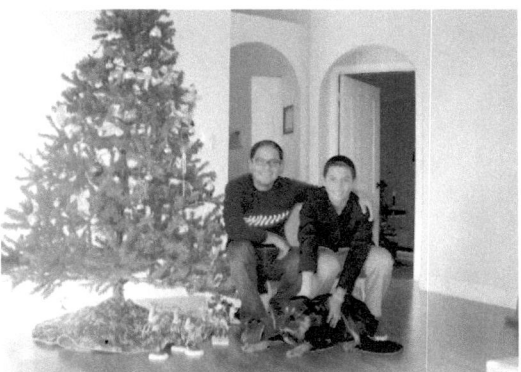

My beautiful boy and me one year before foreclosure.

She wanted me to come and get it. I thought they would bring a container and throw the stuff in there. I felt embarrassed and humiliated. But then I realized I had been irresponsible. I could have done better cleaning the house I had been so graciously allowed to live in. It surprised me because I was expecting to feel anger and a sense of injustice; after all, they had done me wrong. But I was learning to take responsibility. If I'm the problem, then I'm the solution. It was painful, but it was beautiful!

COMFORTABLY INSANE

My sponsor coached me through this time in my life. I was and am so grateful to him and the new people that surrounded me. You see, I was in the program and willing to do whatever it took. But after all the years, at times, I still didn't know what that meant.

> **Lesson Learned:** Accomplishing hard things helped me feel better. But they're no substitute for actual step recovery work. I can still feel depression and fail at relationships miserably after doing hard things.

PART 3

TRUDGING THE HAPPY ROAD OF LIFE

The Legacy

"God, I offer myself to Thee—to build with me and to do with me as Thou wilt. Relieve me of the bondage of self, that I may better do Thy will. Take away my difficulties, that victory over them may bear witness to those I would help of Thy Power, Thy Love, and Thy Way of life. May I do Thy will always! Amen."

—Step Three, *Big Book*

A rocket full of energy without a guide—that's how I felt sometimes. This next part of my life gave me the motor and the guiding rotor that I needed.

I was talking with my cousin Manuel, Meme for short, who was ill with cancer and lived in El Salvador. He had to have a colostomy surgery, which means a part of the colon is removed and an opening is made in the abdomen that allows the stool to pass through to a bag. He explained it as, "I need to carry a bag for my poop to go in." He said they lacked supplies, so he found himself having to reuse the same bag by constantly washing it.

In the past, I had shared the third step prayer of AA with him, though what I was going through was tiny compared to him.

COMFORTABLY INSANE

He said, "You shared that prayer with me, and it gave me hope. Now it's my turn to give you hope. Remember, your dad didn't leave you wealth, but he taught you to work. Use it to build his legacy."

For some reason, that did it. It was as if my cousin had reached inside of my very soul and turned a switch on. I had a new compass in my life.

I understood. That's what needed to happen. I needed to focus on making my dad proud. It switched everything, and just like that, I snapped out of that depression.

As I finished talking with my cousin Meme, we exchanged some more words of love and encouragement before I hung up the phone. He would die a few months later. But after talking to him, I immediately opened a box containing my dad's road bike.

Before my dad passed away, he had bought this red bike to compete in triathlons. When he passed away, he wanted me to have it, and my little sister shipped it out to me. The big brown box sat in my living room for a few weeks because I wasn't quite ready to open it. Talking to Meme helped me decide to enter the Ironman, just like my dad had wanted to do when my brother inspired him. My brother had been struggling with weight and decided he would become a triathlete. This interested my dad, who was very athletic and competetive. He had started to train for and compete in triathlons

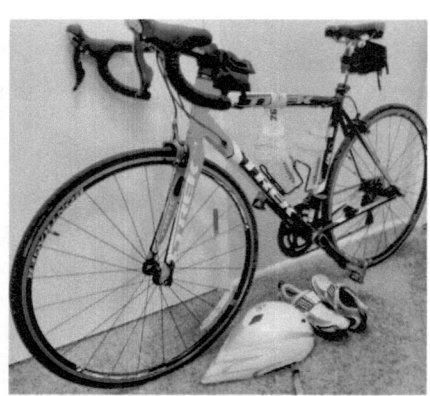

Dad's red bike.

as well, hoping to compete in an Ironman race, which consists of a 2.4-mile swim, 112-mile bike ride, and 26.2-mile run. He actually completed a smaller sprint triathlon in between chemo sessions.

As a family, we had the opportunity to rally in support of my brother in his very first Ironman race, which took place in St. George, Utah. It was a long, arduous race. We coined the term *attack!* and would yell it loud and proud whenever we caught glimpses of my brother. As he finally crossed the finish line, the announcer said, "Mauricio, you are an Ironman!" That was quite a moment for my brother and for us.

Now, it was clear. I needed to complete an Ironman on my dad's behalf. From that point, it took several attempts, but after four years, that's exactly what I did. Maryland Ironman 2016, October 1.

When I crossed the finish line, I thought, *Dad, you are an Ironman.*

Lesson Learned: My Dad left me the tools (a red bike) to find sobriety. He had more wisdom than I could ever imagine.

Amber and Becoming a Lawyer

"And the wheels just keep on turning
The drummers begin to drum
I don't know which way I'm going
I don't know what I've become
For you I'd wait till kingdom come
Until my day, my day's done
Say, you'll come and set me free
Just say, you'll wait, you'll wait for me."

—Partial lyrics to Coldplay's "Till Kingdom Come"

After graduation, I actually landed a regular cushy job. I was very unhappy about it. Haha! Sorry, but I was. It might have been my self-sabotaging "pattern" at work. While I was earning a decent paycheck, I felt trapped and uninterested in the job.

But I thought maybe I just needed to be happy with the good paycheck. After all, in the *Big Book*, I had read some stories of people getting sober and then just living quiet lives without ambitious goals. I thought I would give it a whirl. It was hard, but I did it for just a short while. But I quickly realized a quiet life wasn't for me. I was restless and soon found a new goal!

COMFORTABLY INSANE

I was going to go to law school! The LSAT exam would become my new obsession.

When my bachelor's diploma came, I didn't want to open it. I just let it sit there.

My real diploma was going to be law school, so I didn't need to open this one, or so I told myself. But really I hadn't learned to celebrate success. That diploma represented success, and in a funny way, it depressed and scared me. Ha! My comfort zones. Insanity and failure.

I've since learned that success is to be embraced and celebrated. I love this mind shift.

After four years of trying to find someone to date, I met Amber through a Christian dating site. I figured I would have a better connection there.

I met Amber at a coffee shop one afternoon. I drove my clunky car, which stuck out like a sore thumb in Miami. We immediately connected and talked for hours. I couldn't believe it. We were so different yet the same. Things went so well that it was soon time for dinner, and we decided to drive to a nearby restaurant. She had a really nice car compared to my clunker. For some reason, it seems everyone in Miami has very nice cars, whether they can afford them or not. Heck, I've even seen people delivering pizzas in BMWs and Mercedes.

Anyway, I was proud of my clunker. It was my dad's car. I drove it almost as a badge of honor, so I insisted on going in my car. After all, I wanted to date someone who liked me, not my car. We drove from the coffee place to the restaurant. It was truly amazing. I felt ready! As we drove, it started raining. In Miami, it rains really hard. Guess what. My windshield wipers didn't work. I had to get out of the car and wipe down the windshield, although it made little difference. I was forced to drive very slowly. In my mind, this was perfect. I could be me. I wasn't pretending to be anyone else.

This led to a six-month relationship that shaped my very core in sobriety. I felt I was so mature. And now I was going to be the best boyfriend. I had been in training for four years. Everything was going to be perfect!

Wrong! Instead, I obsessed over the LSAT exam. I studied day and night, at home and at work. I used up all my free time to study. Basically, I studied nonstop and made no time for Amber; I was a horrible boyfriend.

Even though I worked very close to her house, I didn't stop by and visit, not sure why. I knew she wanted me to. I also wanted to. Even with my obsessive study behavior and how I seemed to keep Amber at a distance, there was talk of marriage.

I recall Amber saying over the phone, "Neal, everything you need is right here."

For some reason, I couldn't act upon that, even though I truly felt she was right. Instead I just listened quietly and drove home without stopping by. That year, for Christmas, we spent a wonderful time with her family. They showered me with gifts. I, in return, disappeared for a full month. In my defense, I was studying all this time obsessively or, as I like to call it, alcoholically. I completely isolated myself. Saturdays, I would study ten to twelve hours at the library. It never felt that long to me. And whenever I finished my round of studying, I was astonished and a little scared of my ability to disconnect in such a manner.

I ended up hurting Amber and really destroyed the possibility of a different and special relationship. This was a miserable failure at my first test to develop a real connection with someone in sobriety. I was still a selfish jerk when it came to dating and relationships.

COMFORTABLY INSANE

When I finally took the exam, I called her as soon as I got out, as if not talking to her for almost a month was nothing. She was as tender and reasonable as possible and explained that she had moved on. I was shattered and perplexed. I thought, *after four years of working on myself, I'm still the same. Will I be damaged forever?*

The low I thought I had reached sunk deeper. Another barrel. Again, I couldn't understand how I could feel so bad and still live. The thought *maybe I should just end it all* ran through my mind. But God, who protected me all those years, has never let me play with that idea too much. I had to learn to let go in a healthy way. After almost five years of sobriety, I was still dealing with basic relationship issues. I felt that I was never truly going to learn. And it proved to be true as the next couple of relationships ended in failure, heartbreak, and unhealthy feelings. I was in shock. Again, I thought all I had to do was quit drinking and my life would be perfect. But that was so far from the truth. I seemed to require a lot more molding and learning than I ever imagined. There were more lessons to come.

I was accepted to two law schools. Neither was the one I wanted. So just like that, I dropped that dream, which really confused me. It seemed I had given up so much to be a lawyer, but in reality, the pursuit of law was a cover. Something I could hide behind. That feeling was familiar. Was I starting to pretend again?

I was desperate again after that final conversation with Amber. I remember calling my sponsor in a panic. We decided to meet. My car could barely go a few miles without overheating. So I slowly made my way across the heavy congested Miami traffic, stopping every few miles, just to meet him. It would have been much easier not to go, but one thing I had learned is that I must ask for help. Whatever it takes, I need to get there.

Lesson Learned: No matter how many years and concepts I had learned, I still suffered from skewed perception. I was still able to hurt someone's feelings just as badly as when I was drinking.

The Pattern

"We recovered alcoholics are not so much brothers in virtue as we are brothers in our defect, and in our common striving to overcome them."

—*As Bill Sees It*, p. 167

After one failed relationship after another, I finally learned to connect the dots. I was beginning to recognize a pattern. As my mind cleared, this pattern almost seemed to jump out at me. I could almost touch it. One time it became so clear, I wrote a story about it:

Accept him with all his faults.

She says, "You're an awesome, amazing, and wonderful person. The best I've ever met." He says, "No one has made me feel as good as you, and I'll do anything for you and love you now and always."

Then, one day, he does the unthinkable and incomprehensible: a slow and methodical emotional system shutdown. Little by little, it happens.

The reasons are many, but none can justify the actions. They are close-mindedness one day, inconsiderate comments the next day, disappearing and not calling yet another day, putting other things ahead of her, and showing that he doesn't care. He slowly shuts down, unable to stop, for he hasn't learned how to stop, and yes, it turns out his faults are many.

He cannot understand why because he loves her so!

To his credit, he will not give up, as he knows he must improve.

You see, he just longs to be an acceptable, dependable person for her. No desire to be amazing or wonderful or the best or even awesome. Could she not pressure him with those expectations and instead allow for growth by trial and tribulation?

It requires happy and sad moments alike, but if she can only hold on, he promises happiness will prevail.

This will pass as it always does. Can't she accept him with all his faults?

I safely stored these words away. It was new knowledge for me. It wasn't necessarily about a girl. It was about my feelings, my insecurities, and my withdrawals when it came to connecting with others. Relationships seemed to bring out this pattern in its most vivid form. But I would exhibit this pattern of behavior in all aspects of my life. I knew now that I didn't have to be doomed to repeat it. In one of my many attempts to seek professional help with a therapist, I explained this pattern to her, almost like a list of symptoms. To this day, when I visit a therapist for what I like to call tune-up visits, I give it to them almost triumphantly. Here's what's wrong with me, I claim. Here's what I do in life. Help me prevent this. I've had good responses to this approach. I now know that this is a real situation for me. I train my mind not to repeat this and to see what part of the pattern I'm in. It has been a game changer.

THE PATTERN

The feeling of rejection was one that I seemed to invite into my life. I really don't know when it started, but somehow, I would end up with this intense feeling of being rejected. The pain was unbearable, but now, I've trained my mind to do the opposite. I no longer have to be rejected. Instead, I can be happy. Not under the umbrella of perfection but more under the umbrella of sanity. I no longer fear being sane.

Lesson Learned: As my mind cleared, I found that I could look inward and find and analyze my own faults with extreme self-honesty. This made it easier to talk to a therapist and ask for help with exactly what I felt.

The Gift of Desperation

"Turning negatives into positives has become my new skill."

—Neal Linares

During my recovery, calling the emergency AA hotline at four in the morning was normal. I couldn't bear the pain. I crumbled too easily. I would talk to them for hours. Then, during regular hours, I would call my brother, sister, mom, AA friends, and anyone else who would listen. I'd do anything to distract my mind. I felt that if I let my thoughts take over, my own mind would grab me in a chokehold.

I realized that during all this time in sobriety, I had been desperate. Desperate to fix a marriage, desperate to finish school, desperate to be a better father, desperate to be happy, desperate to find financial security, desperate to find purpose in life, desperate to smile, desperate to connect with someone. Desperation surrounded me.

I realize that if I didn't experience this desperation, perhaps I would not have improved. Therefore, however painful it was, I considered desperation a true and honest gift.

One lonely afternoon, I lay in bed crying and crying. I hadn't cried so much since I had started the journey of sobriety five years earlier. I thought, *I'm destined to live life like this, always being unhappy and losing important people in my life.* It was overwhelming. As I cried and cried, a thought poked at me. I could feel God nearby, almost sitting there, letting me know he was there but also allowing me to feel, to truly feel the inner parts of me. The thought took me to a religious talk I had heard referencing a scripture:

"And if men come unto me, I will show them their weakness that they may be humble; and my grace is sufficient for all men that humble themselves before me; for if they humble themselves before me, and have faith in me, then will I make weak things become strong unto them."

I shot out of bed perplexed! There it was! Another answer! If I asked him for help with my weakness of alcoholism, failed relationships, depression, and incomprehensible demoralization, if I accepted these as my weaknesses, they would somehow become my strengths.

It wasn't over! There was hope!

Now my tears turned to tears of joy, peace, comfort, and serenity. From this experience, I've learned to turn every negative into a positive and to not worry because my weaknesses will become my strengths if I show humility and ask for help.

Lesson Learned: Desperation isn't a bad thing. It can lead you to better things!

Stability in Chaos

*"If you don't spread your wings,
you will have no idea how far you can fly."*

—Unknown

The next couple of years seemed like a blur. I breathed, ate, and slept sobriety, attending as many meetings as I could.

One time, my sponsor said, "Neal, you come to these meetings so you can become a productive member of society. It might be time to be out in the world more."

I had a strong foundation on how to stay sober, but I still clung to the meetings. While I would always need to attend meetings, I knew exactly what he meant. It was time to let go. It felt hard because life was so chaotic. Yet I learned stability in chaos could be achieved.

It was time to let go of the AA rooms and take their messages with me as I became a productive member of society.

Lesson Learned: Even though the ship is sinking, it doesn't mean we're not safe. When the ship is sinking, it's crucial to be levelheaded. After a life of destruction, the sinking ship, in fact, could just be my old life sinking and a new one emerging.

I Count

"I'm no better or no worse than anybody else."

—from AA rooms

When I understood that I could be a productive member of society, that I could reach goals in a healthy way, I felt like a real, valid, legitimate individual. No more pretending. No more pretending not to care. But I still like the song!

I discovered that all those times I said "I don't care" was more a safety mechanism. Actually, I was protecting myself from how much it hurt. Deep, deep down I cared. I just was confused. I learned when you are going through such a transformation or living a life of destruction, you still have feelings. However messed up they might be, you still have them. For me, dealing with the pain, rejection, and everything else confused me. I could not handle this, so it was easier to say I didn't care. Life has taught me that there is an unhealthy "I don't care," as well as a healthy "I don't care." And it all depends what that certain situation makes you feel and true honesty to oneself to know which one is which.

I accepted for the first time in my life that I counted just as much as everyone else. Even if I failed, even if I succeeded, I counted just the same.

Lesson Learned: Put myself in the sphere of validity. My feelings, my thoughts, my life counted. I needed to embrace this so I could become a productive, healthy member of society.

He Made Me.
Build on This Foundation

"He is like a man which built an house, and dug deep, and laid the foundation on a rock: and when the flood arose, the stream beat vehemently upon that house, and could not shake it: for it was founded upon a rock."

—Luke 6:48

I subscribe to the idea that God made me, that He made this world. He has given me my lot in life. Therefore, I'm responsible for it, and no one else. Because of this, I can build my foundation on Him. And that's what I've chosen to do: seek Him for help, ask Him for forgiveness, trust His guidance as it directs me to find open doors in my life, and run away from easy and flashy things, knowing that they are mostly not real. I stay on task to the very end, building my strong foundation.

This allows me to be imperfect. And that seems to be the only thing I can do perfectly!

When I'm at my strongest, I take mental notes and ingrain them deep in my mind. I do this because I realize that one day, I'll be weak. When that time comes, I want to have my mental notes ready.

COMFORTABLY INSANE

I will embody those notes at the right time to give me strength and carry me through because just as every moment passes, I'm sure to experience many more good times and many more bad times. I have no doubt of this. I embrace it. Never do I believe that once a good time has arrived that it will remain forever. As I now know, it too shall pass. On the other side of the coin, the same thing will happen with bad times. They will pass as well. I know this to be true.

My life is my building and creation, and my soul is my foundation that's now resting on the rock of God.

Lesson Learned: God created me. All I needed to do was double down on this belief and foundation, asking and listening directly to Him for guidance as I understood and felt Him.

Back to Basics

"Having had a spiritual awakening as the result of these steps, we tried to carry this message to alcoholics, and practice these principles in all our affairs."

—Step Twelve, *AA*

Life straightened out. I connected with simplicity and humility. During this time, I moved to another small room that I rented from the kindest lady I have ever met. Sometimes, I had to park far away because there were too many cars in this building, but my heart was full of gratitude no matter what.

On the long walks from the parking lot to the apartment, I was grateful I had a roof, food, transportation, and a job. It didn't matter if I didn't exactly like where I lived or where I worked.

All that mattered to my grateful heart was that I had them, and they were true gifts! This kind of gratitude made all the difference.

I honestly felt that I had stopped reaching lows. Before, it felt like each low was at the bottom of that barrel, and then I was always surprised that a new low would come and the barrel was even deeper. But finally, I felt that I had stopped going down, and now I was looking up, standing up, smiling, and feeling good.

I focused on the basics: gratitude, simplicity, God, and letting go.

Lesson Learned: However hard life gets, it doesn't matter because as long as I follow the roadmap of sobriety as laid out in the AA recovery tools, I'll be safe.

The Move

*"We must be willing to let go of the life we have planned,
so as to accept the life that is waiting for us."*

—Joseph Campbell

I had become familiar with the term *geographical relapse*, which meant that someone might move to another city to solve their problems only to find out that the real problem was themselves. Because of this, I refused to leave Florida. I didn't want to feel like I had to escape my circumstances. It was very important. But now I was ready. I felt whole. I felt humble and just wanted to move. It was weird how suddenly my work had an opening in Salt Lake City, my birthplace of all places! I immediately applied. I had talked to my boss before and reached out to the people in SLC. It was super easy how it happened. I was so amazed. I thought that this is how things are supposed to be, and I jumped at the opportunity. After packing up all my things, I left Florida without any chaos and headed to Utah.

My little sister and brother-in-law kindly received me in their home. For years, I had harbored resentment against the state of Utah. Haha! Yup, the whole state! However, I learned through step four that, deep down, the resentment was mostly about my inability to take responsibility for my actions. The state had not done anything to me, but merely reacted to how I had acted.

Regardless, I was nervous to be back; after all, the judge who wanted to put me in juvenile detention had practically kicked me out. I had to remind myself that I wasn't the same person. I was sober. I understood many things now. I had a foundation that I believed in.

Once I arrived, I had to provide lots of papers for work, which included a driver's license. As I sat in the DMV, I had forgotten all the chaos I had caused as a teenager. When they called me up, they informed me I had a $345 pending fine.

Surprised, I asked why.

They explained that I had an unpaid fine from over twenty years ago.

In one second, everything flashed before my eyes. All the arrests, all the divorces, all the failures!

After I paid it, I dejectedly walked to my car and slumped into the seat. I thought, *is my past ever going to leave me alone? Am I ever going to escape the life that I led?*

Then the thought came, *this too will pass. I now have a foundation. There's nothing that I cannot overcome.* I quickly pulled out my mental notes of success, and I let go of the feelings. I was astounded at how quickly I was able to do that.

THE MOVE

Lesson Learned: If my life is in order and I am not running away, moving can be a good thing.

Bliss

"By this time, in all probability we have gained some measure of release from our more devastating handicaps. We enjoy moments in which there is something like real peace of mind. To those of us who have hitherto known only excitement, depression, or anxiety—in other words, to all of us—this newfound peace is a priceless gift."

—*Twelve Steps and Twelve Traditions*, p.74

I loved living in Utah. Even though it was freezing cold, I felt at home. The minor license setback taught me that as long as I was responsible and followed through, things worked out. The universe wasn't necessarily plotting against me. It was, more than anything, neutral and only reacted to my actions.

I continually reminded myself that I was good, that I counted, that I was worth it.

This has changed my outlook on life.

I had reached seven years of sobriety, and for the most part, I felt that elusive peace and serenity I had been wanting, which was a huge contrast to the eight years of white-knuckling it.

COMFORTABLY INSANE

Whenever I drove on the freeway in Salt Lake City, I was always mesmerized by the majesty of the mountains, which were so close. I would play a CD my brother had given me titled "From Here to There" by Paul Martinelli. It consisted of motivational quotes with a soft piano background. It was so soothing. I had kept it and listened to it throughout all my sobriety. In fact, I have listened to it so much that it skips and gets stuck in the CD player. The combination of the quotes and the natural beauty of Utah amplified my feelings of peace and serenity. I was overwhelmed. I cried just about everywhere I went.

And this time the crying didn't come from a place of desperation or incomprehensible demoralization. I didn't feel lost or bouncing around in the bottomless pit of a barrel. I didn't have the feeling of impending doom. I didn't fear not having material possessions or being rejected by anyone. It was the weirdest thing. I felt comfortable in my own skin. Truly comfortable. I cried out of happiness!

I knew I was quirky and not so cool. But that's just who I am. I liked myself.

Therefore, it was so much easier to like others. To be grateful for everything around me. I felt joy for the first time in what seemed to be my entire life.

Lesson Learned: Bliss can be mine!

And Then There Was Amy!

"She took my arm,
I don't know how it happened
We took the floor and she said,
'Oh don't you dare look back
Just keep your eyes on me.'
I said, 'You're holding back,'
She said, 'Shut up and dance with me!'
This woman is my destiny
She said, 'Oh oh oh
Shut up and dance with me.'"

—Partial lyrics to "Shut Up and Dance" by Walk The Moon

The first church activity I attended in Utah was a hike to a place called the "Living Room," which had beautiful views of the Salt Lake Valley. Utah has some of the best scenery—if we could just get rid of the cold. Ha!

At the activity, I met Amy. She is beautiful, fun, and just has this awesomeness about her. We immediately formed a deep connection. The church we attended was comprised solely of single adults. It was just what I was looking for—a chance to meet and date and be friends with a lot of people.

I once had a sponsor who said that "Sometimes, alcoholics don't know how to treat women and much less be in a relationship." He once told me a story of how he gave dating advice to someone he sponsored. It went something like this:

"Okay, I want you to get on a dating site. You're going to set up a coffee date. You'll arrive early. Once your date gets there, you'll greet her like a gentleman. You'll listen to her with both ears and smile. Then you'll say, 'It was a pleasure to meet you,' and the date will be over. You should do this a hundred times. This will help you to learn how to be cordial and treat women right."

I thought it was odd but saw the wisdom in it.

So I took his strategy to heart and dated as much as I could. Meanwhile, my friendship with Amy grew. It always felt so good to be around her. As I dated other women, it seemed I often found myself thinking, *this would be so much more enjoyable with Amy*. After seven months of friendship, we officially changed our relationship and started dating as a couple. The transition was rocky because we were so used to being friends. Now we were dealing with each other on a different emotional level. I could feel the depth of the connection.

It was awkward to make the change, but it was easy to accept that we definitely had a deep connection. We both felt it. I learned how to be more patient and learned that in healthy relationships, it's okay to have a sense of autonomy. We were growing closer and developing an identity as a couple while at the same time learning to be our own people. This was hard for me to grasp at first. I had always believed that you sacrificed yourself fully for the relationship. It was new territory for me, but I was happy to be there. Amy and I soon got engaged and married shortly after.

AND THEN THERE WAS AMY!

It's ironic that I end my book with my own wedding because I made fun of this ending in *novelas*, dramatic Hispanic TV shows filled with passion and betrayal, similar to American soap operas. We had a beautiful wedding in the mountains of Salt Lake City. Her family is amazing, just as my family is.

We had an awesome choreographed flash mob dance at the reception, which had always been a dream of Amy's. Our brothers and sisters and I were so happy to comply! We danced to the song "Shut Up and Dance with Me." I loved it because it felt as if she were literally grabbing my hand and leading me right into the life I had dreamed of having, experiencing peace, serenity, and a strong unshakable connection with her.

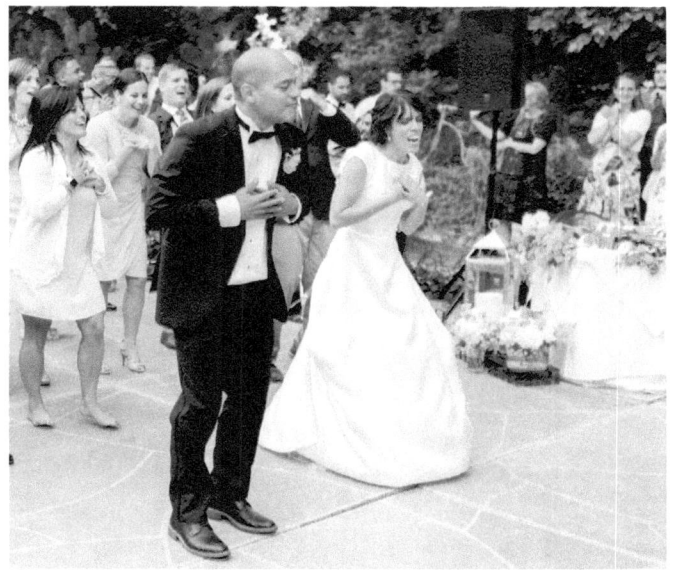

Flash mob dance.

COMFORTABLY INSANE

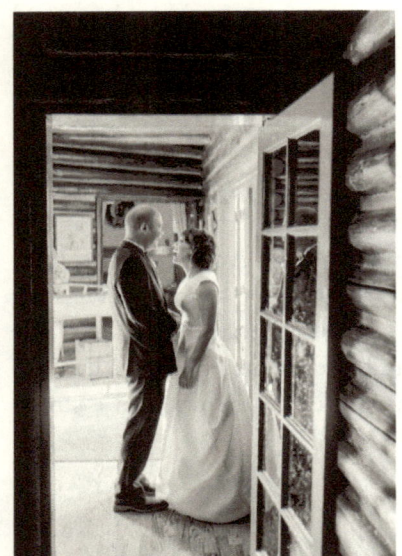

Amy & I right after the cake destroyed news.

It was a great day despite our cake being ruined on the way to our venue. The caterer was in bumper-to-bumper traffic and was forced to slam on the brakes too hard. It was literally in pieces when it arrived. The caterer was so apologetic and almost in tears, but you know what, we didn't even care. We were so overjoyed, it didn't affect us or the night in any way. We were happy.

And we are so happy.

We live in Nampa, Idaho, now. Last year my wife was asked to volunteer at our church as a Cub Scout leader. When they had the pinewood derby event, she invited me to watch. I took my dad's derby car just in case they would let me race. And sure enough, they did. It didn't do so well because with all the moves, the wheels weren't adjusted well. But as you can imagine, to me it was priceless.

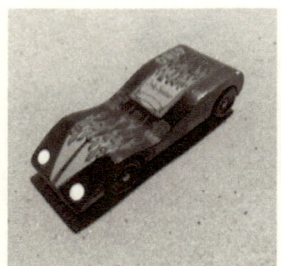 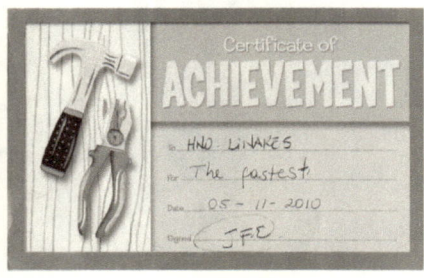

My dad's pinewood derby car and certificate of "The Fastest".

AND THEN THERE WAS AMY!

I have a great relationship with my wife. It's not perfect, but I realize that's okay. I'm able to express with sincere feeling what I can or can't do. I give myself the opportunity and time to think about this deeply so I can let her know. I have found that letting her know how I truly feel is my biggest form of respect and love to her. My wife is an amazing, strong woman. Sometimes she doesn't know her power. But she is learning. We are learning!

Of course, there's work to be done. I keep the AA *Big Book* close by and still attend meetings. As I finish writing this book, I'm coming on ten years of sobriety. The official date is September 28, 2019.

I still have lots of ups and downs and lots of insecurities. But knowing that alcoholism is a disease and that I have it helps me to work things out. I keep strengthening my foundation in every moment, so I can increase in strength.

We live a simple life now, hoping to be blessed with children soon. But we know it's God's will and not ours.

Although things aren't always perfect in sobriety, I've learned that hard things are part of learning.

When I was using alcohol, I felt like life was insane. The reality was that I was insane. Alcohol gave me an excuse to fail, to be crazy. Removing this would make or force me to live life in the normal sphere.

That's what I feared. I feared sanity.

Sanity meant having to be normal. After realizing this, I now understand that no matter what, life is beautiful!

COMFORTABLY INSANE

If you're suffering, I say sanity is the better way. Insanity is what may deceptively keep you safe, but ultimately, it will destroy you just as I was being destroyed.

For today, I'll take another twenty-four hours of sanity. Just for today! Taking it one day at a time.

Lesson Learned: With its ups and downs, I can enjoy life!

Acknowledgments

I never understood what the journey of sobriety meant. The mind shift of insanity to sanity has been life changing. I have so many people to thank, people who have influenced me throughout my life. I am deeply grateful for every encounter, both good and bad.

My AA groups throughout the years have been steadfast. They are my family wherever I am in the world, even on cruise ships!

My parents showed me how to persevere. I'm always reminded of stories of how they overcame many obstacles both in their marriage and in their professional lives that I can apply to my current life.

My beautiful wife inspires and motivates me. Not too long ago, we took a road trip. I was so happy that for the first time in my life, I sang in the car. Of course, she was sleeping. But she seems to know how to let me be me, and I love her for that!

My beautiful son is my driving force. I love you! I'm sorry for not being there 100 percent, but as my dad once said to me very softly, I'm here now.

My brothers and sisters. What can I say? They are all special, and they all rock!

My editor, Katie Chambers of Beacon Point LLC, for picking up the project halfway through and patiently helping me mold my manuscript.

Random Thoughts

To the security guards at juvenile detention centers: know that your words can make the difference in empowering a young person to open up. The biggest tool you have is rapport.

———

To the English teacher: don't blame someone for sticking gum on a chair only because he fits the profile.

———

To the universe: thank you for leveling things out, no matter how bad I got. As long as I did the work, there was always a lesson and good results.

———

To the community service officer: your corruption does nothing to help out kids.

———

To the drunk guy: your advice of paying tithing has been the best advice I have received.

———

To the person claiming to want to learn new things: know you can't learn new things staying in a bubble of your current things.

COMFORTABLY INSANE

To my son: I missed your formative years. You said it doesn't matter, but I know what I didn't give you. One day you will understand. I love you! You're my inspiration!

To those who wrote the anonymous quotes: If I didn't cite your name, I apologize. Somehow, your words came into my life, and I just don't know how.

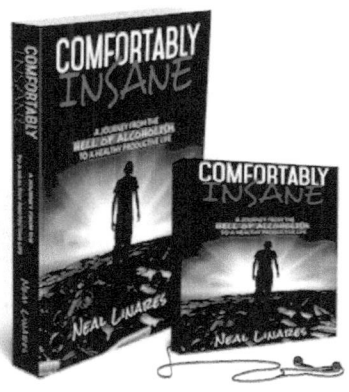

The Number One Question I'm Always Asked Is:

"Neal, Do You Have An Audiobook?"

For a long time I didn't! But finally now I do and the ONLY way to GET it is through this special offer.

Go to: audiobook.comfortablyinsane.com

About the Author

Growing up constantly moving between El Salvador and the US, Neal Linares turned to alcohol at a young age to cope with feelings of loneliness. He found comfort in "insanity," sinking deep into the world of alcoholic addiction. Now having achieved ten years of sobriety, he has felt a burning desire to share his story to both aid in his recovery and to help others with theirs.

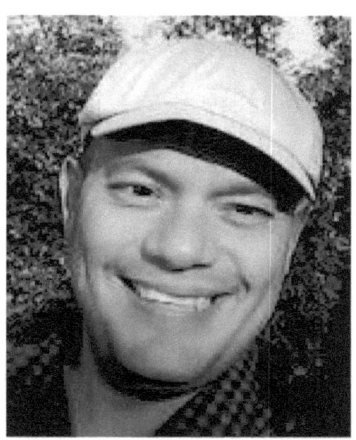

Neal has a bachelor's in business from the Florida International University. When he isn't working on his business endeavors, he enjoys running, training for triathlons, and listening to and working on his relationship with his wife, Amy.

He hopes everyone learns that change is within them. Anyone suffering from an addiction can achieve a spiritual and physical transformation required to overcome their addiction.

Can You Help?

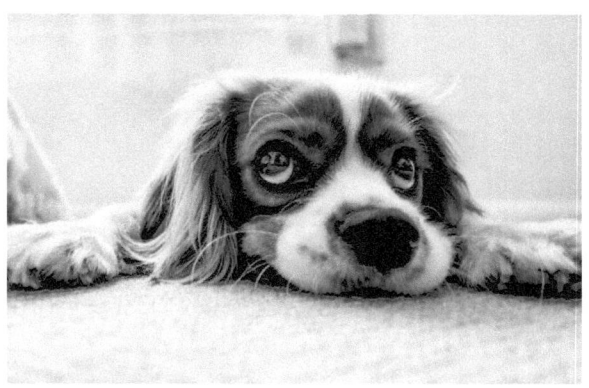

Thank you for reading my book!

I really appreciate all of your feedback,
and I love hearing what you have to say.

I need your input to make the next version
of this book and my future books better.

Please leave me an honest review on Amazon
letting me know what you thought of the book.

Thanks so much!

www.ingramcontent.com/pod-product-compliance
Lightning Source LLC
Chambersburg PA
CBHW020409080526
44584CB00014B/1243